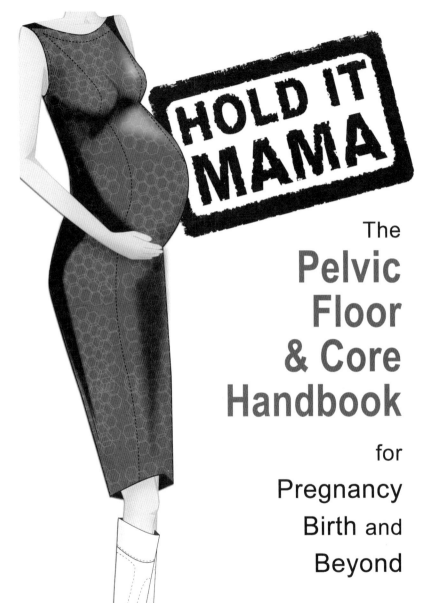

HOLD IT MAMA

The
Pelvic
Floor
& Core
Handbook

for

Pregnancy
Birth and
Beyond

Mary O'Dwyer

HOLD IT MAMA
THE PELVIC FLOOR AND CORE
HANDBOOK FOR PREGNANCY, BIRTH & BEYOND

First Published 2011
Reprinted 2012

RedSok Publishing
PO Box 1881, Buderim, Queensland, Australia 4556
www.redsok.com

www.holditsister.com

ISBN: 978-0-9870766-2-5

Cover Design & Illustrations by Maggie Allingham
Edited by Tania McCartney,
Photography by Barry Alsop, Eyes Wide Open

Printed in Australia by The Ink Spot, Maroochydore

Disclaimer
All names used in the case studies are fictional. This book represents research and clinical experience, is for educational use and is designed to help the reader make informed decisions.

This book is not a substitute for treatment by a physiotherapist or doctor.
The publisher, author and distributors expressly disclaim any liability to any person for any injury or inconvenience sustained, or for any use or misuse of any information contained in this book. The author has made every effort to provide accurate and clear information in the book, and cannot be responsible for any misinformation.

This book is a work of non-fiction. The author asserts her moral rights.

HOLD IT MAMA

The pelvic floor handbook for pregnancy, birth and beyond

From the author of *Hold it Sister!* comes this indispensable guide to the pelvic floor, pelvis and abdomen during pregnancy, childbirth and postpartum.

Physiotherapist and women's health professional Mary O'Dwyer has been treating women for over thirty years and holds a particular professional interest in the pelvic floor. She is an advocate for effective pre-exercise assessment protocols to ensure safer pelvic friendly exercise for women. Mary has undergone postgraduate studies at Melbourne University and is currently a Fellow at Bond University in Queensland.

She conducts practical workshops to empower women with self-knowledge and trains fitness professionals to identify at-risk clients and prescribe safer exercise.

Other books by Mary O'Dwyer:

My Pelvic Flaw (Redsok Publishing, 2007)

Hold It Sister (Redsok Publishing, 2010)–a completely revised and updated version of *My Pelvic Flaw*

holditsister.com

Acknowledgements

This book would not have been possible without my dearest friend and editor, Tania McCartney cheering through ongoing edits despite her own heavy writing schedule; to Maggie Allingham for her stylish diagrams and the sunshine she brings; to Barry Alsop for his humour and professional photos; to Natalie for falling pregnant at the right time; to the lovely Australian and United Kingdom mothers who contributed birth stories, and to the many Australian midwives and physiotherapists for professional reviews. Thank you Craig, Daniel and Sam for reviewing and sub-editing and deepest thanks to my husband Craig for his care and support.

Dedicated To…

Mary Ellen

Mary Bridget

Laura Elizabeth

…for your gifts of grace, love and strength.

Contents

The Pelvic Floor

Pregnancy

Preparing for Labour

Interventions During Labour

Birth

Early PostPartum

Recovery After Vaginal Birth

Recovery After Caesarean Birth

Pelvic Floor Self Assessment

Introduction

Amazing changes in the pelvic floor, pelvis and abdomen occur as pregnancy, labour and childbirth transform a woman's body. Many women and partners have unanswered questions about potential pelvic floor and abdominal issues associated with pregnancy and birth. I've written this handbook for expectant and new mothers to provide practical information and specific solutions concerning the pelvic floor and pelvis during pregnancy, labour, birth and postpartum.

The questions I am most frequently asked, are:

- How do I prevent tearing during a vaginal birth?
- Does caesarean birth prevent incontinence?
- Which positions are best to birth my baby?
- Why are pelvic floor exercises necessary after a caesarean?
- Why is sex painful since my baby's birth?
- How do I know if I have a prolapse?
- Which exercises help separated tummy muscles?
- Why is my caesarean scar still painful?
- Am I doing pelvic floor exercises correctly?

Pregnancy is the ideal time to regularly exercise the pelvic floor to support the growing uterus, maintain continence and control pelvic and lumbar strain. *Find It, Control It, Train It*—my easy-to-follow 3-step program—will help you develop the correct pelvic floor muscle action, strengthen pelvic floor muscles, and learn the exercises which train and protect the pelvic floor throughout life.

During birth, pelvic floor integrity is enhanced through using gravity-assisted positions, pelvic movement, pain management techniques, visualisation and relaxed jaw breathing. Birthing in a calm, safe environment with caregiver and partner support allows women to maintain focused awareness and trust their bodies' ability to birth naturally.

Specific chapters on recovery following vaginal and caesarean births are included. Both vaginal and caesarean births have the potential for pelvic floor and abdominal complications, which clearly benefit from early rehabilitation of muscles and scars.

After baby is born, recovering pelvic floor annd abdominal muscle strength is a high priority. The *Shrink the Jellybelly* routine introduces exercises to improve strength from the inside out, as early as 24 to 48 hours after an uncomplicated vaginal birth. This safe, graduated program works to rebuild and maintain pelvic floor, core and trunk strength.

I hope this handbook increases your confidence during pregnancy, labour, birth and postpartum by presenting preventative measures and treatment options to minimise pelvic floor and associated pelvic/ abdominal risks. At the end of each section you will find a page for writing questions to follow up with your antenatal carer.

Websites have been included throughout the book as alternative sources of information, which may vary between different countries. Always seek the opinion of your antenatal carer before deciding on a course of action.

More than the technicalities involved in birthing and pelvic floor health, my dearest hope is that *Hold It Mama* brings you the confidence, joy, emotional and physical strength every woman should feel on her journey to motherhood... and beyond.

Mary O'Dwyer

A note to the reader:

Always seek professional advice from a women's health physiotherapist, midwife, general practitioner, obstetrician, gynaecologist or urogynaecologist if you are concerned about any pelvic floor issues throughout your pregnancy, labour and postpartum period. Advice given in this book should be considered in conjunction with advice from your healthcare professional. The publisher, author and distributors expressly disclaim any liability to any person for any injury or inconvenience sustained, or for any use or misuse of any information contained in this book. The author has made every effort to provide accurate and clear information in this handbook and cannot be held responsible for any misinformation.

SECTION 1

The Pelvic Floor

Anatomy

The pelvic floor is an intriguingly complex area with a span of muscles, tendons, nerves, blood vessels, ligaments and connective tissues. It contains different muscular layers with strong connective tissue (endopelvic fascia) and external genitals. The muscles sit inside the pelvic girdle bones that join at the pubic symphysis in front and at the sacroiliac joints in the back.

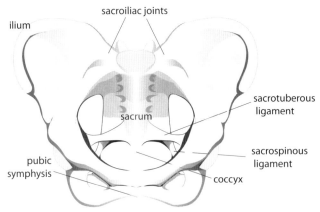

Fig. 1. The bony pelvis

The pelvic floor muscles (PF muscles) attach underneath the pubic bone and join into the coccyx bone at the base of the spine, the pelvic sidewalls and sitting bones. Think of them as muscles with a trampoline-like action providing 'lift and hold' for pelvic organs to close sphincters and prevent loss of fluid, wind and solids. Healthy PF muscles automatically lift before sneezing, running or lifting a weight. This action may not occur when pelvic floor dysfunction is present.

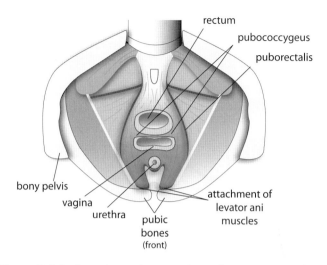

Fig. 2. Pelvic floor from above with urethra, vagina and rectum surrounded by the levator ani muscles.

The Incredible Pelvic Floor Muscles

These 'down under' muscles are unrecognised, multi tasking achievers, thanklessly coordinating various tasks every day of your life. Many women mistakenly believe pelvic floor problems are a normal part of birthing or ageing and are not sure what to do when issues occur. You are about to take a pelvic floor journey, learning how this area works and becoming familiar with your internal pelvic floor.

Understanding the multiple pelvic floor actions will reinforce the need for regular attention to maintain good pelvic health. The role of healthy PF muscles in maintaining continence, preventing internal organ descent, enhancing sexual pleasure, supporting the growing uterus, and working with other muscles to support the spine and pelvis, is discussed below. Healthy pelvic floor muscles automatically lift to coordinate the following actions:

1. Maintain Continence

The muscular complex is designed to close and reinforce the sphincters of your bladder and bowel, preventing loss of fluids, wind and solids with sneezing, lifting or exercise.

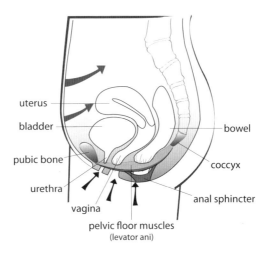

uterus

bladder

pubic bone

urethra

vagina

bowel

coccyx

anal sphincter

pelvic floor muscles
(levator ani)

Fig. 3. Pelvic floor elevation, side view

2. Protect the Spine

The PF muscles don't work alone: they tighten with the deep abdominal muscle transversus abdominis, the deep spinal muscles (multifidus) and the diaphragm. Together, these are the inner core muscles.

Tightening and lifting the pelvic floor automatically co-contracts the core muscles to provide stability to pelvic and lumbar joints. In conjunction with the strong trunk muscles, they support the spine to prevent injury during activity. In some women with PF dysfunction, abdominal muscle contraction causes pelvic floor descent. Retraining the pelvic floor to lift correctly is discussed on page 17.

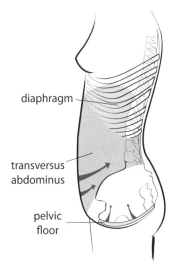

diaphragm

transversus
abdominus

pelvic
floor

The action of pelvic floor and transversus is
to tighten and control internal pressure.

Fig. 4. Core muscles

3. Support Pelvic Organs

The healthy pelvic floor automatically lifts and holds to support the
bladder, uterus and bowel with activity or lifting a weight. Pelvic organ
prolapse occurs when the pelvic organs descend and bulge down into
the vaginal walls. Prolapse is common in women and prevention relies
on practising correct pelvic floor habits and maintaining PF muscle
strength throughout life.

4. Contribute to Sexual Sensation

During orgasm, PF muscles contribute to sexual sensation and the
intensity of muscle contraction. Rhythmic contractions occur in
the pubococcygeus muscle (PC) and other PF muscles along with
contractions of the anal sphincter, rectum, perineum, fallopian tubes,
uterus and vagina. Strong, responsive PF muscles maintain vaginal wall
strength and orgasmic sensation.

5. Open for Childbirth and Elimination

During crowning, as baby's head moves down through the pelvic floor, relaxation without tightening reduces the risk of muscle tearing. Relaxation of the pelvic floor also facilitates full bladder and bowel emptying.

What Causes Pelvic Floor Problems?

It is a common myth that childbirth is the main cause of pelvic floor problems. While giving birth contributes to pelvic floor dysfunction in some women, many other factors contribute to the variety of symptoms that indicate all is not well 'down under'. The main causes of problems and their symptoms are explained in the next section.

Pelvic Floor Muscle Weakness

Signs of weakness include:

- Leaking with sneezing, lifting, exercise (stress incontinence) or orgasm.
- Frequent toileting 'just in case' (this habit trains the bladder to hold smaller amounts of urine).
- Leaking due to urgency with running water or putting a key in the door (urge incontinence).
- Poor control of wind or bowel contents (faecal incontinence).
- Incomplete bladder or bowel emptying.
- Bulging at the vaginal entrance, a heavy, dragging sensation, pelvic or sexual pain indicates the organs have slipped down into the vaginal walls (pelvic organ prolapse).
- Loss of vaginal sensation and orgasm strength.
- Poor posture and altered breathing.
- Chronic sacroiliac and/or lumbar spine pain.

Pelvic Floor Muscle Tightness

Signs of tightness include:

- Bladder urgency and straining to pass urine; frequent voiding and passing small amounts of urine.
- Constipation, straining, anal fissures and haemorrhoids.
- Pain with sexual penetration or insertion of tampons.
- Trigger points in pelvic floor and pelvic muscles.
- Altered breathing and excessive trunk, abdominal and PF muscle tension.

Constipation

Straining to open the bowel progressively damages nerves supplying the PF muscles, causing a loss of bladder and bowel control. Chronic straining weakens bladder, uterine or bowel supports and contributes to prolapse. Delayed or incomplete emptying is typically due to prolapse of the back (posterior) vaginal wall, or failure to release the anal sphincter.

Waist Measurement

Women with a larger waist measurement have a higher risk of pelvic floor dysfunction. Visceral fat accumulates internally around the pelvic organs forcing PF muscles to work harder to support the weighted organs. Visceral fat acts like an endocrine gland releasing chemicals, which weaken the capacity of connective tissues to recover following damage, e.g. after childbirth or pelvic surgery. Overweight incontinent women gain significant improvement when they lose weight. Research shows that a diet high in calories and saturated fat (found in cream, processed meats, fried food) causes a 2.5 times increased risk of incontinence in women. This is possibly due to the inflammatory effect of saturated fat and associated endothelial dysfunction (the layer of cells lining tubes and cavities), which is associated with urinary incontinence.

Heavy Lifting

The internal abdominal pressure created by heavy lifting overwhelms pelvic floor control when the muscles lack quick strength, coordinated lift and hold. If PF muscles fail to lift and hold during heavy tasks, internal supporting ligaments and connective tissues are at risk of being stretched, leading to pelvic organ prolapse.

Pregnancy and Childbirth

Pelvic joints and ligaments are under strain during pregnancy due to the extra weight of baby and amniotic fluid.

Studies show pregnant women are at more risk of developing ongoing postpartum stress incontinence when they experience the following factors: urge incontinence before pregnancy, incontinence during pregnancy, rapid birth or second stage delay, the baby is malpositioned or weighs over 4 kg. A pre pregnancy maternal body mass index (BMI) exceeding 25 is also a risk factor. BMI is a measure of body composition and can be calculated at the following site: nhlbisupport.com/bmi

The use of forceps or ventouse (vacuum extraction) to assist birth is associated with a higher rate of damage to PF muscles and tendons. Just as damaged muscles, tendons and ligaments are rehabilitated after falls, surgery or sport; the pelvic floor also responds to an effective program of strengthening pre and postpartum.

Research shows women who regularly trained their PF muscles at least 3 times a week during pregnancy did not experience more muscle tearing, episiotomy, forceps, suction or risk of an emergency caesarean when compared with women who trained less than once a week. Other studies have found that regular PF exercise increases the size, closing pressure and strength of PF muscles.

Prolonged Abdominal Workouts

The pelvic floor is a smaller muscle group that is rarely trained to counter internal pressure rises and often fatigues during exercise, long before the heart or lungs. The PF muscle endurance required for a long run or prolonged exercise is considerable. Pelvic floor damage occurs when it fatigues part way through a workout. Consistently building abdominal strength with upper abdominal bracing exercises increases intra abdominal pressure that has the potential to overwhelm pelvic floor control.

Repeated rises of intra-abdominal pressure or even one sudden, heavy episode may result in pelvic floor damage, even prolapse, in some women. If continued fast or high-load exercise results in loss of PF and core muscle control, other muscles substitute to provide trunk stability. Over time the body adopts incorrect muscle substitution and altered posture when the PF and core muscles repeatedly fail in their roles of strength and endurance.

Returning to exercise or lifting heavy weights before regaining PF muscle strength, postural alignment and dynamic stability postpartum, results in more strain and damage to pre-weakened muscle, supporting ligaments and connective tissue supports.

Conversely, sustained vigorous exercise (without rest periods) results in increased abdominal and PF muscle tone in some women, causing continued muscular tightness. Poor bladder and bowel control, painful intercourse and some pelvic pain syndromes are related to increased resting tone (tightness) in PF muscles. Muscular overactivity during exercise is avoided by building in regular relaxation breaks, and changing over challenging exercise or training programs.

Prolonged Coughing

Women with chronic lung or respiratory disorders (asthma, cystic fibrosis, bronchitis) or who smoke, have a higher rate of stress incontinence. Quickly lifting PF muscles, described as the 'knack' (see page 21), before coughing helps prevent urine loss and future pelvic organ prolapse.

Weak Connective Tissue

Collagen is the protein in connective tissue giving strength to skin, joints, muscles, ligaments and tendons. Studies indicate when a mother experiences prolapse, daughters have a higher risk of future prolapse (due to inherited collagen types). Hypermobile joints (knees, elbows, fingers and thumbs) that bend too far backwards due to joint laxity and soft tissue elasticity, indicate a higher risk of prolapse following childbirth.

It is important for mothers with hypermobile joints to focus on PF exercises and protective habits, wear support garments and discuss birthing options with their caregivers. For more information: hypermobility.org

Emotional Reactions

Just as some people unconsciously clench their jaw and grind teeth with tension, others unknowingly store 'emotional' tension in PF muscles. When these muscles are constantly held tight, the resulting pattern of excess tension causes bladder and bowel dysfunction and pelvic pain.

Effective treatment involves a program of breathing training, postural control, relaxation techniques, muscle stretches, soft tissue mobilization and specific PF exercises. In addition to treating physical symptoms, professional counselling assists with recognition of underlying causes of tension.

Discovering Your Pelvic Floor and Muscle Action

To become more familiar with this amazing part of your body, start by getting to know your pelvic floor from the outside in. Angle a hand mirror and begin the exploration propped up in bed, sitting on the edge of a chair or in squatting.

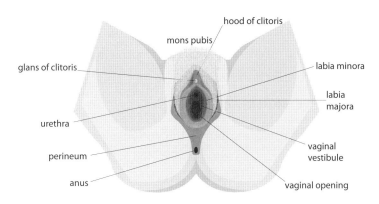

Fig 5. External pelvic floor

Start by locating your mons pubis (covered by pubic hair) and the pubic bone underneath. Move down to your clitoris; drawing back the covering hood will expose the sensitive tip or glans. The thicker, outer labia (majora) are covered with hair; parting the inner labia (minora) reveals the urethral (urine) and vaginal openings. The vestibule is the area surrounding the vaginal opening and the area between the vagina and anus is the perineum.

Vulva is the name given to the area around the vaginal opening, the labia minora and majora and the clitoris. Sometimes, images from powerful fashion and pornographic industries lead women to question their individual and unique body shapes. Just as women have marked variations between feet, breasts, fingers, legs and just about every anatomical area, it is normal for clitoral and labial sizes to range from smaller to larger and vary in colour. Learn more about your internal pelvis with the postpartum vaginal tour on page 133.

Smaller muscles (ischiocavernosus, bulbocavernosus) close the vaginal opening. The perineum is supported and strengthened by the transverse perineal muscle that connects to the deeper PF muscles (levator ani) that lift internally to close sphincters and support organs. An effective PF muscle action closes the vagina, and lifts internally to raise the pelvic floor and switch on other core muscles. This action may need training in women with pelvic floor dysfunction.

Finding Your PC Muscle Action

These five practical tips are ways to learn the effective lifting action by initially observing, and then feeling the correct action of your pubococcygeus (PC). This muscle is part of the levator ani muscle and is involved in bladder control and sexual response. Normally, PC contraction with orgasm stops urine loss during intercourse. The PC has a right and left sided attachment to the back of the pubic bone and along with the puborectalis muscle (which loops around the anal sphincter) joins into the coccyx and lower sacrum. Together these muscles compress the anal, vaginal and urethral openings and lift upwards.

The PC lift is felt towards the front of the pelvic floor whereas the anal sphincter lift (puborectalis) lifts up the back of the pelvic floor. Initially, learn to identify your PC muscle before training it to lift and strengthen with **all** the PF muscles.

Find which of the following actions helps you recognise the internal lifting action of your PC muscle. I have included a training activity after each item to improve awareness of this muscle in action. Use self-examination as a chance to become more familiar with how your pelvic floor works. The following exercise skills are important for pregnant and postpartum strengthening and every day PF muscle control.

1. Mirror Mirror

Sit on the edge of a chair and angle a mirror to view your pelvic floor. Part the labial lips and observe what happens with PC lifting (while breathing out), as though trying to slowly stop the flow of urine. You should see closing and a slight lift of the urethral and vaginal openings. The anal sphincter draws in, but focus the lift to the front of the pelvic floor with thighs, buttocks and waist relaxed.

Do this again and focus on a slow closing and lifting of the urethral and vaginal openings. Observe the floor relaxation when letting go of the lift.

Now watch what happens to your pelvic floor when you cough strongly. If it bulges down, the PC and other muscles are either weak or slow to respond. This may also happen during activity or exercise when it should tighten and lift. Failing to correct a faulty pattern of pelvic floor descent leads to incontinence and pelvic organ prolapse. If the floor 'holds' when coughing, your PF muscles tightened at the right time.

Activity: Become aware of tightening and lifting the pelvic floor before you cough or lift. Learn the PC lift and repeat this action when standing, walking, coughing and lifting. While this may be initially difficult, keep practicing until it becomes a more familiar action.

2. Tampon Tug

Wash your hands before swelling a tampon with warm water and inserting vaginally. Try to keep the tampon in place while pulling slowly on the string. If the tampon holds and you need to pull more firmly, this indicates your PC is tightening. If the tampon pulls out easily, then the muscle lacks effective strength.

Activity: Insert the tampon, gently pull on the string, tighten and lift vaginally to hold the tampon in place for 5 seconds. Relax and repeat 5 to 8 times. Remove the tampon after use.

3. Hold it Sister

This activity is not an exercise, but a way to help identify the sensation of using your PC muscle. Try to slowly stop the flow of urine during bladder emptying but only try this occasionally, as the bladder should empty in a continuous stream.

Activity: Try this action no more than once a week, as a measure of muscular control.

4. Feel for Yourself

Insert your index and middle fingers about an inch inside your vagina. Repeat the PC lift to feel squeezing and drawing-up around your fingers; this is the correct action of the muscle. A healthy muscle feels full and firm around the fingers whereas a weak muscle feels soft with less response. A variation in muscle size and squeeze pressure between right and left sides may be noted. If nothing happens or the lift is minimal, the muscle is weak or damaged, or you don't understand the lifting action of the muscle.

Move your fingers higher and sweep them around the upper vaginal walls, which are quite capacious. When you feel a central firm 'dimpled chin' you have located your cervix. During labour, the cervix dilates fully to form a continous birth canal from uterus to vagina.

If inserting fingers is difficult or painful, this indicates PF muscle tightness or a type of vulval pain syndrome.

Activity: If muscle tightening is absent or the insertion is painful, consult a gynaecologist to exclude pathology or disease and visit a women's health physiotherapist for treatment and management advice.

5. The Right Vibe

Vibration gives increased sensory input to muscles. Many women have discovered the benefits of using a vibrator to reach orgasm, but less known is that vibration increases a muscle's ability to contract, improving its strength.

If you use a vibrator, insert it vaginally (with a little lubricant), and tighten your PC around the vibrator. A definite closing and squeezing action around the vibrator should be felt.

Activity: Insert the vibrator and repeat PC tightening and relaxation, holding for 5 to 10 seconds and relax before repeating. If your PC fatigues (the tightening action becomes difficult), take a break to allow for muscle relaxation.

The 3-Step Program - Find It, Control It, Train It

There are three stages to this program—finding the correct PC muscle action, strengthening the PF muscles for daily activity, and training the muscles to cope with exercise or lifting.

Find It

The **Find It** exercise teaches three things: firstly, how subtle the PC action is. Secondly, how to lead the pelvic floor lift with the PC muscle, and finally, how the PC muscle works with other PF and core muscles (transversus abdominis, deep spinal multifidus and diaphragm). If you are confidently lifting the PC after practicising some of the previous practical actions, this section will be easy to follow.

PRACTICAL SESSION

- Sit tall and lean forwards to rest forearms on your legs, with bottom well out behind in the chair. If you normally hold your waist drawn back, practice abdominal wall release by placing a hand over your stomach and feeling the softening release of muscle tension.

- Breathe in slowly and deeply, expanding the base of your ribs and breathe out continuously through pursed lips.
- On the next long out breath, imagine slowly drawing a tampon back in vaginally. This is a *slow, gentle* movement, starting from underneath the body, to feel the PC action without other muscles jumping in first. Hold this tension and breathe to avoid breath holding.
- Feel how your urethra and vagina close and lift slightly in an upward direction.
- If this PF muscle action is difficult to feel in sitting, try side lying for easier stomach relaxation. Move back to sitting when you feel confident the action is correct.

If you struggle to identify the muscle action, try a different mental cue. Imagine a sharp needle coming towards your urethra and vagina. Slowly close your urethra and vagina and lift up internally away from the imaginary needle as you breathe out continuously through pursed lips.

The lifting action feels like a gentle urethral and vaginal lifting (this is your PC muscle) along with firmness at the bikini line and perhaps lower back. This second sensation is the transversus abdominis and deep spinal core muscles tightening with the PF muscles. *You are now feeling how the PC lift connects with the tightening of core muscles.*

Hold for 5 to 10 seconds as you breathe. Relax the pelvic floor and repeat 5 to 8 times. Repeat this action at least three times during the day. *If you can only hold the PC lift for a few seconds, aim to gradually increase the length of hold with further practice.*

Some women find their PC muscle 'flickers' initially. With practice, this flicker gradually becomes a sustained muscle hold. Many of my clients say they 'hardly feel anything' and this is normal to start, as it's a slow, gentle lifting sensation in this early learning stage. The PF muscle action is very different from what you feel when tightening a strength muscle. It's like the difference between lightly squeezing the tip of the index finger and thumb together, compared with making a strong fist.

Forget about strength during the **Find It** stage, as this learning has nothing to do with strength. It is about locating and coordinating the muscles in a gentle manner, so your brain learns the correct action without stronger abdominal, chest wall, and buttock or thigh muscles dominating.

Only after confidently locating and lifting the PC from underneath the body, should you start to internally lift these muscles more firmly. The next stage is about improving strength with five to six months of regular PF exercises.

Control It

I hope you are gaining new respect for your PC. It is a remarkable superstar muscle, working across the whole spectrum of activity from slow to fast, from gentle to strong, and deserves daily attention.

If your PC is tightening correctly in sitting and standing, it is time to progress exercises and build pelvic floor control into everyday activities.

PF muscles experience three levels of strength and endurance:

- The PF muscles stay constantly switched on, at a low-level, during the day when you are sitting or walking tall. This is **low-level endurance**.
- The PF muscles combine strength and endurance for sustained load activities—for example, with fast walking uphill or carrying a child. This is **strength endurance**.

- The PF muscles react rapidly with any sudden, unexpected loading—for example, sneezing or tripping. This is **quick strength**.

As the pelvic floor has multiple actions, three separate training exercises are required to prepare your muscles for different daily activities.

Exercise 1: Endurance

Every morning, begin with the low-level **Find It** exercise to reinforce the correct lifting action, and then advance the technique with a little more endurance training.

While sitting or standing, grow tall and relax waist tightness. As you breathe out, draw up the PC and hold this light lift for 10 to 30 seconds, while continuing to breathe. Repeat this light lifting action during the day.

Activity: Grow tall through the crown and feel the PC and deep abdominal (core) tension automatically switch on. Improving postural control is the *easiest and most effective way* to keep the low-level endurance of your PC switched on.

> Try this simple test to feel the effect 'growing tall' has on your PF muscles. Sit on the edge of a chair with attention on your pelvic floor. Feel what happens to the pelvic floor when you fully slump, and then what happens when you grow tall through the crown of your head. Try this action again and feel the pelvic floor 'give way' with slumping and lightly firm with the tall posture. Without consciously lifting your pelvic floor, growing and staying tall does this for you!

Exercise 2: Strength

Start this exercise in forward sitting, with a relaxed waist. While breathing out, lift your PC and continue lifting up higher and higher vaginally, along with squeezing and lifting your anal sphincter. Hold and breathe for 10 seconds. Relax completely for 5 to 10 seconds, and then repeat 5 to 8 times.

This is a stronger internal lift, so keep focused on deep vaginal internal lifting, and feel all the abdominal muscles start to tighten together. If dizziness is felt, too much effort is being used.

Progress the exercise to standing. Place both hands on a table, lean forward and stick your bottom out behind. Tilt your bottom up, lengthen through your crown, relax the waist and soften the knees. This position helps you isolate and start the lift from the front of your pelvic floor. Also try this exercise on hands and knees with forehead resting on forearms or sitting on the floor in a crossed-legged pose.

Activity: Pelvic floor descent with exercise weakens internal bladder, vagina and bowel supports. A good test of pelvic floor functional strength is keeping the PF lifted while standing up from a squat. Train your PF muscles to lift before and hold during the movement, as squatting is an everyday action.

Exercise 3: Quick Strength (The 'Knack')

To ensure your pelvic floor reacts quickly when coughing, sneezing or jumping, practice this third exercise. In forward sitting, quickly and strongly lift your pelvic floor internally as before, hold for 2–3 seconds, and then relax completely. Do 8 to 10 of these quick, strong internal lifts and rest when the muscles fatigue.

Activity: Repeat quick lifts to train an early pelvic floor response to sudden movement. Try quick pelvic floor lifting and holding with simulated coughing to practice this exercise, first in tall sitting then in standing.

Training Routine

Commit to a regular training routine with all three exercises to develop endurance, strength and quick strength.

Start by repeating each of these exercises three times a day, starting with five and increasing to 8, then 10 repetitions per session.

- To gain more benefit from the strength exercises, practice them in different positions—sitting, kneeling on all fours with head down, open-leg sitting—then progress to forward-leaning standing and upright standing.
- Challenge the PF muscles more as you improve, by adding a second set of exercises after a 60–second rest. Feel the sensation of your PF muscles 'letting go' in between exercises.
- *Using a vibrator or biofeedback probe provides a resistance to the internal squeezing, lifting action (review vaginal exercisers on page 150). Practice pelvic floor tightening around your partners erect penis during intercourse for exercise and feedback.*
- PF muscle strengthening takes around 5 to 6 months for most women, although many notice gains after 2–4 weeks of training. After the initial training period, continue with 1 set of exercises most days of the week to maintain strength throughout life.
- Incorporate the PF lifting action into daily activities for a lifetime of pelvic floor control.

If PF muscles are tight and difficult to relax, or you have pain, only do Exercise 1, and seek the advice of a women's health physiotherapist.

Activity: Repeat these exercises daily for 30 days to ensure they become part of your health routine. Stick a calendar on the bathroom mirror or wall and mark off each day of practice. On completion of day 30, you are officially a pelvic floor athlete!

The Protective Bracing Pattern (PBP)

Maybe you have decided to start exercising after giving birth or wish to lose weight and tone up. Great planning goes into organising exercise clothes, the best sports shoes and regular times to exercise. Probably, the last thing considered is how exercise could affect your pelvic floor!

If occasional leaks have you avoiding certain exercises or activities, learning to switch on the pelvic floor and abdominal muscles *together* will enable you to progress your exercise program. The **protective bracing pattern (PBP)** provides this final link.

PRACTICAL SESSION

This final exercise starts with identifying what happens to your pelvic floor and abdominal muscles with coughing.

Sit upright with waist relaxed; push both hands firmly into the sides of your waist. Cough strongly and feel the waist widen out sideways under your hands.

Now repeat the same action again and note what your *pelvic floor* does during the cough.

If your pelvic floor also lifts (or firms) and holds during the cough, then the PF and core muscles are automatically tightening together, as the outer abdominal muscles brace. This action of pelvic floor lifting, with the front abdomen flattening and side waist widening, is your body's **protective bracing pattern (PBP)**.

If the waist narrows under your hands, the abdomen bulges to the front or your pelvic floor pushes down, then the floor is not coordinating with other core and abdominal muscles. Retraining the floor to lift while all the abdominal muscles tighten is now a priority. Go back to learning the gentle pelvic floor and deep core action, as well as the quick strength exercises for rapid pelvic floor lifting with simulated coughing.

The final step to total pelvic floor coordination is learning the PBP as an exercise, as a strong, coordinated PBP protects your bladder against leaks, prevents prolapse and supports the spine during exercise or lifting. Learning this action provides an understanding of the *control* needed with exercise rather than pushing your body to perform difficult tasks.

If the pelvic floor descends or the abdomen bulges out during gym exercise, stop the activity, and choose an easier option.

Activity: Sit upright and push both hands firmly into the sides of your waist. Make a strong, long 'hissing' sound and feel the waist widen out into your hands. Stay tall to avoid bending forwards at the waist.

Repeat this action (staying tall), lift up the pelvic floor first, and feel the waist widening with the strong 'hiss'.

When the pelvic floor lifts and holds with waist widening, you are doing the PBP as an exercise. Always lift from the pelvic floor *first* when repeating this exercise. Notice the difference between your abdomen flattening and widening at the side waist compared to the incorrect action of sucking in the navel and crunching forward (to flatten the abdomen).

Hold the PBP exercise for 5 to 10 seconds; relax and repeat 5 to 10 times. Repeat this same action in standing.

Practice the PBP daily to strengthen this newly acquired pattern and start integrating this action with exercise and daily activity.

If you do not understand or experience difficulty with any of these exercises, please consult a women's health physiotherapist before continuing to the next stage.

The PBP is similar to but different from the pushing action used when your body takes over pushing during labour. The labour pushing action is the same action as used to empty the bowel.

To practice the birth opening action, feel your waist widen with the long 'hissing' sound and this time, push the lower abdomen forwards with relaxation and opening of the pelvic floor. Bowel emptying and birth are the only times this action is used.

Train It

Once you have mastered the pelvic floor lift and integrated the PBP, start training your pelvic floor as part of a total body program. The exercises from page 163 show examples using various positions, apparatus and movements to train all postural muscles, leading with the pelvic floor.

Start the exercises at a slow, even pace, and always focus on tall posture to maintain the PF and core action throughout the whole exercise. If you cannot maintain the PF lift or the load or speed of movement is too much, back off a little and work on control.

As your pelvic floor coordinates and strengthens, increase the level of resistance of bands or weights, increase the speed of movements or add to the complexity by standing on a stability disc. Relax PF muscles between exercises, re-engaging them before repeating the movement.

After 16 weeks of pregnancy, avoid lying on your back to exercise. Begin the seated, then standing exercises, and engage the PBP before the exercise. Refer to Exercise in pregnancy on page 40.

Start by practicing the first five exercises 2 to 3 times a week and add another exercise each week.

SECTION 2

Pregnancy

Managing Your Core and Floor During Pregnancy

While many women sail through pregnancy, others experience aches and pains as their body transforms. The body has nine months to adapt, but during the later months, changes in weight distribution stress the pelvis, spine and supporting structures. Typical pelvic/abdominal conditions include separation of the outer abdominal muscles (diastasis rectus), sharp abdominal twinges, pelvic heaviness, low back and scaro-iliac pain, leg or vulvar varicose veins, constipation and haemorrhoids. This section contains information on how to manage and alleviate conditions affecting the pelvis, abdomen, spine and pelvic floor, to improve your overall pregnancy and birth experience.

Bladder Control

Pregnancy is the first time some women experience bladder leaking. The sphincter muscles controlling the 'holding in' of urine are softened by pregnancy hormones-progesterone and relaxin, reducing their firm closure. In early pregnancy these normal hormonal changes plus increased blood flow to the kidneys cause bladder frequency and increased urine production. Some mothers are prone to urinary tract infections in the early stages of pregnancy, while in later pregnancy; toilet trips are more frequent due to uterine pressure on the bladder.

The bladder is pushed forward by the uterus and loses some of the angle at the bladder neck needed for closure and continence, so leaking may occur. To reduce the likelihood of bladder leaks, start PF exercises early in pregnancy and continue after baby is born. Always use the lifting 'knack' action before coughing, sneezing or lifting (see page 21).

Research information reinforces the importance of controlling leaking during pregnancy.

- Studies show regular PF exercises during pregnancy decrease postpartum urinary incontinence.
- Bladder leaking before or during pregnancy increases the risk of being incontinent after baby is born.
- Weight gain during pregnancy is not associated with increased urinary incontinence, however failure to lose weight gains six months postpartum *is* associated with incontinence.
- Results from one study show intensive PF muscle training during pregnancy seems to facilitate rather than obstruct labour, and could prevent a prolonged second stage in some women.
- Frequent toilet trips are normal during pregnancy. Before pregnancy the bladder usually empties five to six times a day and once at night.
- Weak bladder control responds well to a committed PF exercise routine, tall posture and support garments.

If you suspect a urinary tract infection:

- Increase water intake, avoid caffeine and use urinary alkalinisers if frequency, burning or back pain develops. Visit your doctor if you feel unwell or if symptoms persist beyond 24 hours as ongoing infection can lead to more serious kidney infection.
- To control an urgent bladder (no infection), lift the PC muscle, curl toes under and breathe slowly for 10 seconds or until the sensation fades. Do not restrict fluid to control urine loss.

Pelvic Girdle Pain

The pelvic girdle transmits weight between the upper and lower body and maintains dynamic trunk stability through balanced posture and synergestic muscle action. Pregnancy weight gains, centre of gravity changes, strenuous work, previous injury, increased BMI, hormones, daily postures, exercise habits, position of baby, and quality of the connective tissues affect the stability of the pelvis.

As pregnancy progresses up to 33 per cent of women develop varying degrees of pelvic girdle pain (PGP), pelvic or pubic symphysis instability. All of these terms refer to pregnancy-related pain and instability of the pubic symphysis (front of pelvis) and sacroiliac joints (back of pelvis) that may or may not be associated with low back pain.

Stabbing, shooting, dull, or burning pain focuses around the sacroiliac joints, one or both buttocks, back of legs and pubic bones. Walking, twisting, and stair climbing are painful. Sometimes a clicking or grinding is felt in the pubic bone making walking difficult after standing. The discomfort is worse at night lying on the back, turning over in bed or lifting legs to get out of bed. Women with combined low back and PGP suffer more disability, often needing a walking stick or crutches to stay mobile.

Studies of pregnant women with PGP show they have dysfunction in their PF muscles, indicating specific PF muscle training is a crucial component in gaining relief of this condition.

To manage pelvic girdle pain:

- Avoid sitting with crossed legs, on the floor, or in the yoga lotus pose. When the pubic symphysis is painful, avoid straddle stretches or bike riding, which further opens the joint.
- Wear a support garment, or a sacroiliac belt (above the pubic bone) to decrease sacroiliac joint movement. Wear it to bed if pain disturbs your sleep. If the belt increases PGP, loosen it and seek treatment.
- Side-sleep with pillows to support the abdomen and upper leg.

- Squeeze knees together to roll out of bed or get out of the car.
- Improve posture by growing tall and lengthening through the top of the head. Regularly realign working and daily postures.
- Choose upright chairs with a cushion for lower back support; keep a cushion in the car to support the lower back curve.
- Lift the pelvic floor before coughing or sneezing, and stay upright instead of bending forwards.
- Avoid strenuous work and heavy lifting, eg: carrying bags of groceries or an older child.
- Avoid lying on the back for sex; try a side-lying position. When PGP is severe, sex is too painful.
- Wear low-heeled shoes (no higher than 3–4 cms) to reduce strain on the low back, pelvic and leg joints (associated with wearing higher heels).
- Avoid exercises that involve bouncing or balancing on one foot.
- Sit to pull on underwear, socks and trousers.
- Use massage and local heat to relax tight muscles.
- Sleep on a sheepskin for comfort, with a pillow between the knees.
- Seek treatment of PGP to learn postural control and lumbopelvic stability exercises.

Low Back Pain

Low back pain differs from PGP with pain focused in the low back above the sacrum. It is similar to non-pregnant low back pain with restricted low back movement, pain on forward bending and tenderness over spinal muscles and ligaments. Low back pain that is severe or does not settle requires further investigation. Protect your spine and avoid lower backache during pregnancy with the following suggestions.

- Adopt a tall posture when sitting, standing and walking to regain the gentle low back curve, and continue to hold the position.

- Check sitting posture at the computer. Choose a chair that supports thighs with weight evenly distributed on sitting bones under the buttocks. Stand and move about frequently. Check chair height and optimal computer positioning on the desk. ergonomics.com.au

- Engage in gentle exercise such as walking, swimming, tai chi, pregnancy yoga or aqua natal classes to ease spinal discomfort (modify the exercises if you have PGP).

- Exercises prescribed to non-pregnant women with back pain are modified for pregnancy.

- Stop strenuous daily activities and heavier lifting, particuarly in a forward bent, twisting action to avoid excessive strain on low back and sacroiliac joints.

- Bend both knees to lift; keep a straight back (bottom out with chest lifted engages strong spinal muscles), and use the 'knack' to lift PF muscles (see page 21).

- Exercise pelvic floor, core and abdominal muscles regularly to reduce and control low back pain.

- Wear a support garment. The BellyBra is a full torso support undergarment designed to provide gentle support for the lower back and abdomen after 26 weeks. A wide elastic band sits below the tummy to support the weight of the baby while the back stretch panels support the spine and improve posture. bellybra.com

- The newer SRC support garment provides support and compression to the pelvis, pelvic floor and thighs, while supporting the hips and lower back. A reinforced gusset helps to compresses vulval varicosities. recoveryshorts.com.au

- Wear shoes with a lower heel to avoid the pelvis from tilting further forwards. Foot discomfort is related to baby and maternal weight gains. Additonal pressure on supporting structures under the foot lowers the arches, adding to their length and width. Regular foot massages and orthotics arch supports bring relief.

- Use heat or ice packs and massage to alleviate spinal muscle tension. Side-lie for massage when the baby bump prevents lying face down. Some clinics provide a special pregnancy table to accommodate a pregnant tummy.
- To reduce low back pain, relaxation, massage, stretching, joint mobilization, improved body awareness and specific lumbo-pelvic stabilising exercises are effective measures.

Diastasis Rectus

Diastasis rectus abdominis (DRA) is a midline split of the rectus abdominis muscles at the linea alba, which commonly occurs during mid to later pregnancy. The central linea alba anchors all the abdominal muscle layers and widens as baby grows. The gap usually occurs around the umbilicus but can spread upwards to the sternum or lower to the pubic bone.

Researchers report that as pregnancy progresses, 27 per cent of women develop a separation, rising to 66 per cent in later pregnancy. It is more common in multi-parous, multi-birth, caesarean and non-exercising mothers and associated with back pain and pelvic floor dysfunction.

Back pain and altered postures occur as the separation reduces the abdominals ability to stabilise the trunk. Prolapse, stress and faecal incontinence later in life are associated with a DRA, so protect the abdominals from excessive strain during pregnancy.

Avoid the following actions to reduce midline strain:

- Traditional abdominals—sit ups, crunches, double leg raises.

- Pilates exercises with neck/trunk flexion holds e.g. the '100s' exercise, plank holds, push ups.
- Fitball curl ups or backward stretches over the ball.
- Some yoga poses e.g. wheel and boat poses.
- Lifting or carrying heavy objects e.g. furniture, toddlers.

To protect the midline:

- Wear an abdominal support.
- Hand-support the sides of the abdomen, pushing them together just prior to sneezing or coughing.
- When getting out of bed, roll onto one side and push yourself to sitting before standing.
- Lift the pelvic floor to switch on core muscle support.

Review and practice the safe way to use your abdominal muscles during the pushing stage of labour (page 80) to prevent rectus tearing.

Pelvic Heaviness

If pelvic floor supports were stretched during previous pregnancies or damaged during an earlier birth, they will not be as effective in supporting the uterus during subsequent pregnancies. When the uterus sits lower in the pelvis, feelings of vaginal or pelvic discomfort and heaviness, genital swelling and urine loss occurs. To manage pelvic heaviness:

- Visit your caregiver to determine if pelvic organ prolapse is present. Refer to prolapse self assessment on page 132.
- Fit a vaginal pessary support to reduce pelvic organ prolapse.
- Wear a support garment.
- Continue regular PF muscle strengthening.
- Avoid heavy lifting or standing for long periods of time.
- Try swimming for exercise (water supports the heavy uterus).

Braxton Hicks Contractions

Uterine tightening can begin around 20 weeks and signals the uterus is practising for labour. The contractions vary from light to firm, are usually irregular and last from 20 seconds, up to 2 minutes. During a contraction feel the uterus tightening and firming under your hands. Use the contractions as an opportunity to relax and breathe until the tightening passes. Change activity, take a warm bath, rest and see your caregiver if contractions becomes regular or intensify.

Abdominal Ligament Pain

Supporting uterine ligaments lengthen as the uterus increases in size. The round ligaments are located along the upper side of the uterus and extend down through the inguinal canal (groin) to attach into the labia majora. As the uterus grows, the ligaments are stretched out like a rubber band. Sudden movement can strain the ligament and irritate nerve fibres, causing sharp pain.

Common signs of round ligament pain include:

- A sharp stitch-like pain, on one or both sides of the groin or abdomen. Sometimes a longer lasting dull ache persists.
- Pain on one or both sides of the lower abdomen with fast walking, sneezing, getting up quickly, or rolling over in bed.

Ease abdominal ligament pain by:

- Sitting for a few minutes to reduce strain on the ligaments.
- Changing positions in bed. Try lying on the side without pain and use a small pillow for support under your abdomen.
- Taking a warm bath or applying a hotpack to the abdomen.
- Exercising more slowly at lower intensity; stop heavy tasks.
- Wearing an abdominal support garment.

Seek medical advice if any sharp pain is prolonged or intense.

Constipation

Constipation at some point during pregnancy is commonly due to:

- Reduced fluid or food intake aggravated by nausea.
- Loss of fluid due to vomiting.
- Some medication, painkillers, iron supplements or over-use of laxatives.
- Low fibre diet.
- Slower intestinal movement due to hormonal changes and pressure on the rectum from the heavy uterus.
- Decreased activity.

To prevent straining:

- Increase water to 6–8 glasses a day.
- Increase dietary fibre with extra fruit, vegetables, beans and wholegrains.
- Add soluble fibre, e.g. mix 1 to 2 teaspoons of psyllium husks into a large glass of water or juice twice a day, to bulk and soften the bowel contents.
- Place a stool under your feet, lean forward and relax the abdomen when emptying the bowel. (Fig 6). For the bowel opening action see page 25.

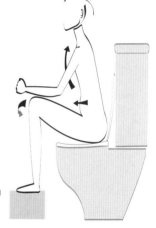

Fig. 6. Toilet Position

- Walk daily for 30 to 45 minutes as exercise improves the movement of the intestinal contents.

Haemorrhoids

Haemorrhoids are caused or aggravated by bowel straining, and are more common in pregnancy due to the marked increase in the body's circulating blood volume. Placental hormones cause relaxation of all blood vessel walls. Haemorrhoids are essentially swollen or inflamed varicose veins in the lower rectum or anus, and can be:

- Internal—these haemorrhoids are painless and identified by light bleeding after the bowel empties. When an internal hemorrhoid prolapses, it protrudes out of the anus after the bowel empties, and is usually painful.
- External—discomfort is felt after the bowel empties and bleeding occurs if the vein breaks. These external veins are painful when swollen. Review treatment of haemorrhoids on page 113.

Anal Fissures

About 10–15 per cent of women experience anal fissures during pregnancy or postpartum. Straining to pass a hard stool, severe bouts of diarrhea or anal sex (less commonly) may tear sensitive anal tissue during pregnancy or after childbirth. Stretching the anal sphincter and mucosa beyond its limit causes a fissure or chronic ulcer in the anal canal. Bowel emptying is extremely painful with light bleeding afterwards.

Increase water and fibre intake, use stool softeners, and adopt the forward leaning toileting position. Wash or wet wipe the anal area after emptying and apply a baby barrier cream, paw paw ointment, corticosteroid or steroidal creams to heal the fissure. Physiotherapy treatment with laser or ultrasound can improve fissure healing.

Vulvar Varicosities

Vulvar varicosities are varicose veins in the vulva that distend and pop out due to pressure of the heavy uterus and altered blood flow to the area. The swollen veins cause pelvic heaviness, throbbing, aching or itching sensations. Once baby is born, the varicosities usually disappear.

To gain relief try the following suggestions.

- Avoid prolonged sitting and standing by regularly changing position and exercise to prevent pelvic blood from pooling.

- Wear a support garment (SRC garment with full leg) to support the pelvic area and abdomen. Compression garments or tights compress leg veins to help them work more efficiently. Put the garment on early in the day to prevent blood pooling in the legs and feet. Adding a thick pad inside firm underwear provides supportive pressure on the varicosity.
- Regularly contract PF muscles to pump blood through the area.
- Take regular rest periods, lying flat for 10 to 15 minutes several times per day.
- Sleep more on your left-hand side to prevent prolonged pressure on the large vena cava vein on the right side of the body.
- In severe cases, the varicosity is injected with a saline solution to collapse it.

Varicose leg veins are common in pregnancy, as the valves (which prevent blood from flowing backwards) don't always work efficiently. When the valves fail to open and close effectively, blood pools in the veins, causing purple, red or blue/black lumpy veins. Office bound mums can develop swollen ankles from continuous sitting and benefit by regularly standing, taking a short walk, one or two short lying down breaks with legs elevated, wearing compression tights and avoiding crossed legs.

If a painful, red, swollen, warm area suddenly develops in your leg, call a doctor for an immediate appointment. An ultrasound will reveal if the pain is due to deep vein thrombosis (blood clot in a leg vein), requiring immediate treatment.

Posture During Pregnancy

As the body's centre of gravity alters, the spine aligns to adopt a new position. It's easy to lose contact with balanced posture during pregnancy, as several factors affect spinal alignment. The heavy uterus changes the body's centre of gravity and pregnancy hormones act to soften ligaments in preparation for birth, causing joint 'looseness', which decreases normal pelvic and spinal stability.

In response to the shifting centre of gravity, the pelvis tips forwards and the pubic bone moves backwards.

The internal supports for the pelvic organs are loaded by the weight of the heavy uterus. Some trunk and hip muscles are overworked and become tight or develop spasms. The abdominal muscles lengthen and are less effective in supporting the lower back and spine if they separate at the midline. Towards the end of pregnancy, it becomes harder to maintain good posture by the end of the day.

Switching on PF and core muscles before activity helps to provide much needed pelvic and spinal support.

PRACTICAL SESSION

Take a look at your body standing with bare feet apart, front on, then side-on in a long mirror. A malaligned posture occurs with abdominal sagging and an excessive inwards curve in the low back. To compensate, the upper body leans backwards and the head pokes forwards. This position concertinas the spine causing aches and pains.

Watch what happens to your lower back when you lift up the inner foot arches, and grow taller through the crown of your head.

Lengthening through the spine relieves spinal joint pressure and engages the PF and core muscles to hold the tall position.

Keep the abdominal muscles engaged and practice the 'growing tall' posture until it becomes a habit; you will find it is worth the effort to relieve low back ache and provide pelvic organ support. Adopt the tall posture when you walk and avoid standing still for too long. Place one foot on a low footstool during a standing task (alternate feet), to reduce pressure on pelvic and spinal joints.

The choice of chair greatly influences sitting posture. Choose a straight-backed chair, push your buttocks into the back and grow tall so the body weight rests down through the sitting bones and lightly under the front pubic bone. Lounge chairs with a raised head support place your spine into a 'C' curve position that brings on spinal discomfort.

Sit in a straight-backed dining chair or on a birth ball to avoid slumping, which pushes baby into a posterior lying position (their spine facing your back).

Slumping or sitting with crossed legs scrunches the front of the abdomen. To encourage optimal baby positioning prior to labour, sit tall to maintain space in the front of your abdomen or lean forward, knees apart, with a straight back.

Uncross your legs and keep both feet flat on the floor with knees apart to prevent low back strain and pressure on leg veins.

Try this activity: lengthen through your crown and place two fingers over your chest bone and another two on your pubic bone and draw an imaginary line between the 2 spots. During the day keep this line from shortening with regular spinal lengthening.

Sex During Pregnancy

Often, new parents have questions about the safety of sex and the effect of pregnancy on their sexuality. There will be changes in your sex life, however understanding, humour, creativity and communication ensures partners remain intimate during pregnancy. Sexual activity and intercourse during pregnancy is normal so long as it doesn't cause pain or discomfort, there are no physical complications, and you want to have sex. Amniotic fluid supports and protects your baby (a bit like bubble wrap on a parcel), so sex does not harm your unborn baby.

Oral sex is safe so long as your partner does not have a cold sore around the mouth or blow air into your vagina (there is a rare risk of causing an air embolism). Anal sex is not recommended during pregnancy for it's potential to transfer infection-causing bacteria from the rectum to the vagina.

If you feel overwhelmed, tired and nauseated during the first trimester, then it's not likely you will feel like sex. Often, the second trimester is when libido returns, as nausea disappears and you feel more inclined to become intimate. By the third trimester, some women experience joint discomfort and feel too exhausted or large to contemplate sex, whereas others report having great sex right up to their due date.

After 16 weeks choose alternative positions to lying on your back during intercourse. Sitting on top of your partner or using the side lying, face-to-face position lets you control the depth of penetration and avoids partner weight on your abdomen. With pelvic girdle or lower back pain, choose a position such as side lying with a rear approach, so your pelvis is supported and comfortable (wear a support wrap and pretend it's a garter belt!).

In fact, sex is sometimes recommended to encourage overdue babies.

Many hospitals use a synthetic form of the prostaglandin found in semen to induce labour when women go beyond their due date. Caregivers may recommend sex close to the baby's due date to naturally start labour (Italian doctors call this an Italian induction), so don't be surprised if this is prescribed to help start your labour.

Intercourse should be avoided when vaginal bleeding is present; there is a history of premature labour, part of the placenta covers the cervix (placenta previa), the cervix is dilated, the amniotic sac surrounding the baby has broken, labour has started or infection such as herpes or other sexually transmitted disease is present. Be guided by your caregiver if sexual activity is contraindicated.

Exercise During Pregnancy

The American College of Obstetricians and Gynecologists (ACOG) recommends that women with low-risk pregnancies participate in moderately intense physical activity for 30 minutes or more daily, on most days of the week. If you are enjoying a problem-free pregnancy, and regularly exercised before pregnancy, continue to exercise but *modify the intensity*.

An expanding abdomen changes the body's centre of gravity, so it's normal to feel less steady and slow down after 24 weeks. If you experience pain or conditions that prevent you staying physically active, seek early caregiver advice, as it is important to learn ways to keep moving throughout pregnancy.

Moderate exercise during pregnancy builds endurance in supporting muscles, making it easier to counteract your body's changing centre of gravity. Even light exercise pumps the heart faster, oxygenates body tissues and organs, stretches muscles, manages weight gain and helps with birth preparation.

Suitable activities include walking, swimming, cycling, prenatal yoga, belly dancing, easy fitball exercises, Tai Chi, light weights and gentle exercise classes. If you are about to start an entirely new exercise routine during pregnancy, consult caregivers for advice and guidelines.

Marked changes occur in the cardiovascular and respiratory systems during pregnancy. Moderating activity or sport avoids overexertion and overheating, and prevents sharp rises in heart and breathing rates.

The heart works 30 to 50 per cent harder during pregnancy, and the number of breaths taken per minute increases, especially after 28 weeks. Use the 'talk test' to monitor exercise intensity. If you can still talk while exercising, you are working at an appropriate level. Not being able to talk due to fatigue or 'shortness of breath' indicates the intensity is too high. Adjust the exercise level lower or rest before recommencing at reduced intensity.

Use a heart rate monitor or manually check the heart rate during exercise (with finger tips over pulse points), to follow the research guidelines below for recommended heart rates during exercise.

In fit pregnant women:

Ages 20–29, 140 to 160 BPM (beats per minute)

Ages 30–39, 140 to 156 BPM

Ages 40+, 125 to 140 BPM

In lower fitness level pregnant women:

Ages 20–29, 129 to 144 BPM

Ages 30–39, 128 to 144 BPM

A balanced exercise program for pregnant women includes the following types of exercise.

Aerobic

Walk, swim, belly dance or cycle for lung and heart fitness and weight control. Exercising in water supports the weight of the uterus, reduces the risk of joint and pelvic floor strain, prevents overheating and relieves swelling due to the effect of water's hydrostatic pressure.

Changing from land to deep water running in a pool allows runners to continue impact free running and prevent pelvic floor and joint strain.

Strength and Balance

Prenatal yoga, modified Pilates, seated fitball exercises, lighter weights and stretch band exercises improve and maintain muscle bulk and strength, while challenging balance control. These activities focus on slow controlled movement to strengthen PF and core muscles, both during pregnancy and after baby is born. Review suitable exercises on page 163.

If you did not exercise regularly before pregnancy, start with an easy activity such as walking, 4 or 5 days a week for 10 minutes, gradually increasing the time up to 30 minutes.

Running after 16 to 20 weeks pregnancy is too challenging for pelvic floor supports (due to hormonal changes in collagen and connective tissues), and runners are advised to walk or deep-water run to avoid strain. Runners and athletic women train their bodies to develop tight muscle tone. Labour and birth proceeds more smoothly for athletic women when they have practiced abdominal and pelvic relaxation (with reverse PF exercises) and perineal massage.

Exercise Precautions

When exercising, remember to:

- Wear comfortable, supporting footwear for ankle and arches.

- Stretch slowly after exercise, but not excessively as pregnancy hormones increase ligament and tendon flexibility.
- Avoid bursts of high intensity or strenuous exercise and lower the intensity as pregnancy progresses.
- Avoid bouncing activities; wear a supportive sports bra during exercise.
- Wear a support garment to reduce PGP, and avoid exercise with body weight on just one leg.
- Avoid lying on your back to exercise after 16 weeks.
- Eat healthy carbohydrates before exercising and sit down if you start to feel light headed. Take some juice or fruit with you to refuel during or after the session.
- Stop exercising if tired or fatigued; pregnancy is not the time to overdo activity.
- Avoid overheating by exercising in the early morning, indoors, or in water (below 30 degrees Celsius); stay cool and drink plenty of water. Position yourself near a fan during a group exercise class.
- Avoid lifting heavy weights, especially overhead in later pregnancy. Strength training with light to moderate weights should be individually assessed.
- Take a break from contact sports during pregnancy or sports with a higher risk of falling such as touch football, hockey, skiing and horse riding.
- *Avoid sit-ups, curl-ups or strenuous abdominal exercises to prevent more stretching on the rectus abdominis muscle midline.*

Avoid aerobic exercise if any of these conditions are present:

- dizziness, severe anaemia
- severe joint, pelvic or abdominal pain
- uncontrolled type 1 diabetes, thyroid disease, serious respiratory

or cardiovascular disorders (exercise can prevent or reduce elevated blood pressure and swelling, especially with a water based exercise program)

- uncontrolled high blood pressure, pre-eclampsia (related to increased blood pressure and protein in the urine)
- incompetent cervix, placenta partially covering the cervix
- under-developed foetus, multiple foetuses
- premature labour, cramping, pre-term rupture of membranes or leaking fluid, vaginal bleeding
- sudden swelling of ankles, feet or hands, morbid obesity

For information on exercise guidelines during pregnancy: acog.org/publications/patient_education/bp119.cfm

Pregnancy

Key Points

- Stay active with some activity most days of the week.
- Exercise in water is ideal right through to late pregnancy as the growing abdomen is supported.
- Use the 'knack' (page 21) to tighten PF muscles before coughing, sneezing or lifting.
- Regular PF exercises are essential to control or prevent bladder leaks and support pelvic organs.
- Increase water and fibre to keep stools soft and avoid bowel straining.
- Sit tall and avoid slumping on the couch to discourage baby from adopting a posterior birth position (with baby's back towards your spine). Sit in an upright dining chair.
- Swim and kneel on hands and knees to exercise as this position encourages optimal baby positioning for labour.
- Prevent constipation related haemorrhoids and anal fissures by drinking soluable fibre in water daily.
- Avoid lying on your back to exercise after 16 weeks and prevent pressure on the large vena cava vein.
- Avoid exercises that widen the abdominal muscle separation e.g. sit-ups, curl-ups, ball back bends, and some pilates and yoga exercises.
- Wear a support garment to add compression to pelvic joints and abdominal muscles.
- Sex is sometimes recommended to encourage overdue babies. Many hospitals use a synthetic form of the prostaglandin found in semen to induce labour when women go beyond their due date.

Pregnancy questions to ask antenatal caregivers

SECTION 3

Preparing for Labour

There are various ways to prepare for labour and birth—ways to gain an enhanced outcome for you, baby and your body longer-term.

Planning is important, as giving birth is hardly a diary note to be scheduled into a busy life and dealt with when the time comes. To ensure the best results, athletes and performers train consistently before their events. Gain the pre-training benefits for labour and birth by developing a similar commitment to practising effective birth preparation skills during pregnancy.

Practising some of the following activities alone and later with your partner will help to physically and emotionally progress labour. Not all of the strategies will suit you. Find a few that are suitable and practice them mentally and physically as you prepare for your baby's birth.

Visualisation

Visualisation is dreaming about the future by creating the desired images of what you would like to happen. Use visualisation to create images of joy, confidence and happiness during pregnancy and birth. Visualisation develops focus on a pleasant scene or memory to distract attention when uterine contractions become more powerful. Many wonderful pregnancy visualisaton CD's are available to build confidence, courage and focus during labour and birth. The following suggestions may help to create your own guided visualisation.

Recall the sense of peace felt while relaxing in a scented bath, floating in a pool or being entranced by the colours of a perfect sunset. Become aware of how mental calmness brings slower breathing, muscular relaxation, inner body awareness and focus.

Step 1

With eyes closed, find your own peaceful image or place—maybe a perfect starry sky or a beach at sunrise. Breathe and become part of this place, where time stands still. Stay with the image and feelings when external noises interrupt. Return to this image regularly, when sitting at a desk, standing in a queue or listening to relaxing music.

Step 2

In *Birthing From Within*, Pam England suggests holding an ice cube on the palm when you are feeling relaxed, to challenge your ability to remain relaxed. Repeating the ice cube test teaches the skill of staying relaxed and focused on your visualization and breathing instead of shifting focus to the sensations produced by the ice cube. Staying fully present with a peaceful image in the presence of an uncomfortable sensation is an important skill to learn before labour.

Practising this skill will greatly benefit your ability to reduce muscle tension and use contractions during labour to help your body give birth. Becoming fearful, breath holding and tightening muscles is counterproductive and slows labour. In *Birthing Skills* Juju Sundin (with Sarah Murdoch) takes readers through her Birth Skills classes in a step-by-step guide of easy-to-learn, proven pain management skills.

Towards the end of my third pregnancy, having finally gained some well-earned birthing wisdom, I sat by a small ocean bay where dolphins visited. Closing my eyes I imagined a sleek dolphin coming to me at the waters edge. I recreated the freedom and wonder of this visualisation during my pregnancy, both seeing and feeling the dolphin drawing me through the water as I held onto its dorsal fin.

When my uterus contracted more forcefully as labour progressed, I imagined the dolphin diving down, taking me under the water and back up again when the contraction passed. I even had the ability to breathe under water and covered a few kilometers dolphin diving through labour!

With my first baby, I was unprepared for labour and had no knowledge of how I wished to birth, let alone my birthing rights. I was placed on my back, feet in stirrups, and given pethidine along with an episiotomy. With subsequent births, focused visualisations and self-directed choices allowed me to connect with and trust my body's ability to birth, resulting in drug and intervention free labours.

Perineal Massage

Research shows women giving birth for the first time can reduce the risk of muscle tears and stitches by practising regular perineal massage in the last four to six weeks of pregnancy (it does not always prevent tearing). Perineal massage lets you experience some of the stretching sensations felt during the crowning stage of birth when PF muscles are under maximal stretching pressure during the passage of baby's head.

Perineal massage has two benefits: it increases the extensibility of PF muscles before labour, and you learn PF muscle relaxation under stretch, in preparation for when baby's head applies strong opening pressure to the floor. Muscles and tendons are more at risk of tearing when the muscles suddenly contract against a stronger force.

Keeping the pelvic floor open during the full stretch by the crowning head (while the uterus contracts with a powerful downwards pressure) is a significant part of reducing the risk of perineal tearing.

Practice the following perineal massage techniques or ask your partner for help, if you both feel comfortable. Seek midwife advice if you are unsure or require further instruction.

- Wash hands and trim thumb nails.
- Relax in a warm bath or apply hot towels to relax the PF muscles.
- Apply cold pressed oil or a non-petroleum based lubricant to the perineum (the area between the vagina and anus).
- Massage while squatting on a low stool or propped up in bed. Place both thumbs about 3 to 4 centimetres into the back of the vaginal opening, just above the perineum.
- With thumbs hooked inside the vagina, slowly stretch down towards the anus and out to each side until you feel a stretching, tingling sensation. This opening action stretches the skin and muscles in a similar way the baby's head stretches them during birth. Avoid the urethral opening during massage.
- Feel yourself 'letting go' as the perineum is stretched, rather than reacting by tightening and closing the PF muscles. Breathe with a relaxed jaw.
- Initially hold the stretch for 30 seconds then relax for a minute. Lengthen the stretch time (and stretch intensity) up to 90 seconds over the next few weeks. Repeat several times twice a day after 36 weeks of pregnancy.
- Do not perform perineal massage if herpes or other sexually transmitted diseases are present.

The Epino device is an alternate method of PF muscle stretching, using a contoured, silicone balloon inserted vaginally and pumped up to slowly hold a sustained stretch on the pelvic floor. In trials, the first time mothers who used the Epino after 37 weeks showed a significant reduction in the rate of PF muscle tearing, compared to the control group of mothers who did not use the Epino device: epino.com

Body Massage

Massage during pregnancy reduces stress, eases spinal aches and pains, relaxes tight muscles and reduces swelling in arms and legs. It gives emotional support, reduces anxiety and the need for medication. Ensure the masseuse/masseur is a therapist with a certificate in pregnancy massage, as some regular massage techniques should be avoided during pregnancy. Massage is not advised during the first trimester of pregnancy. Check with your caregiver before commencing massage sessions.

Belly Dancing

Belly dancing, or 'oriental dancing' began with Middle Eastern women who practised from childhood to prepare them for childbirth (and to discover their sexuality). In the early stages of labour, slow, rhythmic hip circles and figure-eight movements help the labouring woman stay more comfortable. As the intensity of contractions builds, stronger side-to-side or shimmy movements are used to position the baby and relax the pelvic floor.

Women belly danced in a circle around the labouring mother to calm her with swaying movements and encourage her to copy their slow rhythmical actions.

Some women find belly dancing controls back pain throughout pregnancy and helps to regain postpartum tummy control. Belly dancing teaches vital connection and awareness of PF and core muscles. When performing slow, controlled hip-circling movements, different PF muscles rhythmically tighten. Faster hip and shimmying actions involve a higher level of lift and hold in pelvic floor and core muscles. Fast footwork should be avoided during pregnancy to prevent the risk of falling.

Western women generally don't learn pelvic and hip movement. Dance involving pelvic movement while controlling the upper body (and vice versa), is a powerful workout for core and abdominal muscles. Traditional abdominal exercises (lying on the back) build strength in the upper abdominal area; where as dance with pelvic movement focuses on building PF and core muscle strength and endurance in an upright position. Belly dancers maintain pelvic floor and core muscle control with tall upper body posture during hip circling and shimmying moves.

Try this fun action taught by many belly dance teachers. Imagine holding a pencil in your vagina and enjoy the sensation of using your pelvic floor and core abdominals while moving your hips. Stand tall and prevent the pencil from falling out during slow hip circles, both clockwise and counter clockwise. Imagine drawing circles and figure of eights with the pencil. One midwife told me she advises women to write their names, including crossing 't's and dotting 'i's with their pencil action!

See Resources for more information on pregnancy belly dancing DVDs.

Squatting

Squatting helps to strengthen thigh muscles before labour and open up the pelvic area. Practice the squatting action during pregnancy with a fitball (use a pillow if no ball) behind the back, against a wall. Avoid squatting too deeply, as the emphasis is on learning to hold the position and build up strength in thigh muscles, rather than how low you can squat.

- Start by wall squatting with a ball or pillow behind your back for 10 to 15 seconds for 5 repetitions and gradually increase the time held for up to 60 seconds for 2–3 repetitions. Breathe normally during the hold.
- Hold onto a bench or rail and fully squat if you are free of joint

pain: hold for 30–60 seconds and repeat 4–5 times. Practise relaxing and opening PF muscles during the squat, then closing and lifting PF muscles before standing.

- After 34 weeks, sit on a low padded stool with knees wide apart to stretch leg and pelvic muscles.
- If PGP or vulvar varicosities are present, start in a mini squat position with knees together for 10 seconds.

Hypnotherapy

Hypnotherapy with a specialist practitioner teaches essential relaxation skills, visualisation and meditation to assist with a natural, drug-free birth. Learning can be one-on-one, with a class or a home CD. Regular practise with your partner is a way of reducing fear and anxiety and is a method for achieving deep relaxation and training the mind to ignore pain sensations. Hypnotherapy helps to focus your energy and awareness for a more positive birthing experience.

Childbirth Classes

Women learn about pregnancy and labour from a variety of sources such as books, internet sites or by talking to family and friends. Valuable and often vital, up to date information is gained through attending childbirth classes at a local birthing centre or hospital. Some internet information and books can be misleading for your situation or the information may relate to another country. Discuss web information with caregivers.

Childbirth classes are specifically designed for women and partners to learn and ask questions about pregnancy, labour, birth positions, interventions, postpartum care and parenting. These classes may be the only time your partner hears information about birthing and parenting. It's also a great way to meet other couples and develop relationships that continue after baby is born.

Many different organisations run classes, and childbirth educators come from a variety of educational backgrounds such as doulas, midwives and physiotherapists. Classes should cater for the various options women and their partners may choose or face, regardless of where or how they give birth. Educators are most effective when they offer classes flexible enough to suit your needs and don't impose personal beliefs on labour and birthing. Often, the information varies between educators, so ask or shop around to find a suitable class. Ideally, commence the first class early to allow enough time to attend all classes.

Topics covered should include:

- Prenatal development, diet, physical and emotional care during pregnancy.
- Precautions during pregnancy and premature labour.
- Different choices for birthing and interventions used.
- What to expect during labour and birth.
- The role of birth partners.
- Breathing and positions to assist birth.
- Pain relieving techniques and pain options.
- Developing a birth plan and knowing your birthing rights.
- Addressing fears about childbirth.
- Information on unexpected outcomes.
- Breastfeeding information.
- Pelvic floor management and exercise program.
- Advice on early parenting with caring for baby, baby massage and sleep techniques.

Research information on 'active birthing' and labour to help optimise your birthing experience. See resources for active birthing books.

Birth Plan

There are obvious plans to make before having baby, such as organising care for older children, freezing meals in advance, and transportation (and route) to the birthing centre or hospital. Organise a network of family and friends to help with cooking, shopping, housework and babysitting to give you time to catch up on sleep or the freedom to enjoy activities with partners or older children.

Another important step is learning about the risks and benefits of different types of births and interventions used, exploring all options and knowing your rights, including informed refusal. Some women like to write a birth plan to express their wishes during birth.

Consider if writing a plan is a need to intellectually control birth, or an opportunity to determine what is important to you during labour and *ideally* how you would like it to progress, along with procedures you want to avoid. The plan is not a legally binding document but it does inform caregivers about your wishes.

Birth is unpredictable and may completely differ from the plan you have written, so it is important to stay open and flexible to accommodate the unexpected. Keep the plan concise as hospitals are busy places and caregivers are not likely to remember your specific birth plan or read through many pages of information. Some hospitals and caregivers have their own procedures and practises, which override birth plans. Do your homework on the birthing facility and caregiver's policies (during pregnancy) to help with the important decision of where to birth.

Schedule times to discuss the birth plan with caregivers before labour to determine their level of support, and sort out fears or misinterpretations. Ask for the items you agreed upon to be placed into your chart that goes to hospital. Even though the birth support team understands your wishes, keep in mind that birth can occasionally go in unexpected directions when interventions are introduced.

Birth plan items include:

- Your name, age and birth status (e.g. 1ˢᵗ baby).
- Name of birth partner and their role.
- Anyone else you wish to be present for the birth e.g. a doula.
- Atmosphere e.g. dim lights, if you wish to play your own music or use an electric aromatherapy burner.
- Props e.g. ball, stool, own pillows or other comforts.
- Birthing tub/shower—whether you wish to use water for pain relief (tubs are not available in many hospitals).
- Special needs—if you require a specific diet, have religious or cultural needs or a disability requiring special equipment or access.
- Pain relief—what types of relief e.g. acupuncture, Tens.
- Preferred birth positions—whether you want to kneel, stand or lie on your side.
- Assisted delivery—your decision about the use of forceps or ventouse (only used for emergency situations), induction of labour and intravenous fluids.
- Monitoring your baby—eg: midwife with a handheld monitor or using electronic monitor initially, only for a short period.
- Episiotomy—ask caregivers if they do routine episiotomies.
- Placental delivery— if you wish to avoid premature cord clamping and examine or keep the placenta.

Elective Caesarean Birth Plan:

With a planned caesarean or belly birth, think about how you can personalise the birth to ensure a happy, memorable experience. In consultation with caregivers your plan might include:

- Playing your music or asking for a calm, minimal noise environment in theatre.
- A running commentary from the midwife during surgery.
- If you wish the midwife to hold a mirror to watch baby's birth.
- Opportunities for taking photos or video of the birth.
- Placing baby onto your chest for immediate skin-to-skin contact and wrapping in one of your baby blankets.
- Assistance with breastfeeding to establish early contact.
- Consider delayed cord clamping or a lotus birth (placenta remains connected with baby).
- Keeping partner and baby with you for ongoing bonding and emotional support.

Preparing For Labour:

Key Points

- Practise focused visualization and relaxation to develop confidence, courage and focus for labour.
- Enjoy body massage with a pregnancy masseuse to reduce stress, swelling in arms or legs, and relax tight muscles.
- Hypnotherapy with a skilled practitioner teaches relaxation and visualization skills to help you progress through labour.
- Practise slow belly dancing to develop pelvic floor and core control.
- Practise the squatting action to strengthen thigh muscles and sit on a low padded stool after 34 weeks to stretch leg and pelvic muscles.
- Attend childbirth classes with your partner to learn about pregnancy, birth, and postpartum and early baby care.
- Research birthing practices and policies in prospective hospitals and birthing centres.
- Write a birth plan with your partner and discuss with all caregivers.
- Personalise an elective caesarean birth plan to ensure a happy, memorable experience.
- Ask about caregivers birthing practices and policies.
- Engage a midwife or doula to assist with pregnancy preparation, birth and postpartum recovery.
- After 34 weeks ask caregivers how baby is positioned.
- Practise perineal massage after 36 weeks to increase PF muscle extensibility, especially for first time mothers.

Preparing for Labour questions to ask antenatal caregivers and birth plan notes:

SECTION 4
Interventions During Labour

Becoming well informed about labour helps you and your partner decide the best course of action in conjunction with caregivers' advice. Sometimes interventions are required for the safety and well-being of both mother and baby. Interventions should not be routinely used during birth but reserved for emergency situations. Common interventions are discussed in this section, while the following section provides strategies to improve pelvic floor outcomes.

Monitoring

Cardiotocogram (CTG) is used to keep track of baby's heartbeat and your contractions, however studies show it does not necessarily make birth safer. It produces a graphic record of the response of the foetal heart to uterine activity, as well as information about its rate and rhythm. While it benefits a high-risk birth, CTG can limit a woman's ability to move, to use the shower or bath and increases the likelihood of having a caesarean birth. It is usually done externally with leads attached to the mother's abdomen or occasionally an internal monitor is used when necessary. CTG is difficult to avoid in hospitals where its use is policy with syntocinon or epidural injection. Some hospitals now use **telemetry,** which allows the mother to carry a radio controlled device and stay free to move around while baby's heart beat is monitored.

With a syntocinon free birth the mother is able to change positions and move about. The foetal heart is monitored by listening with a handheld **Doppler** machine. If electronic monitoring is used, ask if it is necessary, for how long it is needed and for time off the monitor. Unless syntocinon is used, CTG should only be used initially for 20 to 30 minutes and not left on throughout the entire labour. For more information on foetal monitoring: childbirth.org/articles/efmfaq.html

Pain Relief

An **epidural** anaesthetic involves injection of medication into the space around the spinal cord via a thin catheter between the lower vertebrae, causing numbing from the injection point downwards. Also called a spinal anaesthetic, it is an effective pain control strategy and may also be used to progress contractions if established labour slows due to pain, fear or exhaustion.

The benefits of an epidural must be balanced against a range of side effects: it increases the likelihood of having an episiotomy, forceps, vacuum extraction or caesarean section. As there is little feedback from the pelvic floor, it is difficult to know when to push and less likely a posterior facing baby will turn. When an epidural is used, babies that were previously lying in the anterior (normal) position are more likely to rotate to the posterior position during labour. Posterior presentation produces more stretch on the pelvic floor, increasing the risk of stretch related injury.

Research shows many women who received an epidural experienced a longer second stage of labour and their contractions needed to be stimulated. Some experienced very low blood pressure, were unable to move for an extended period after the birth, developed a fever and had difficulty passing urine.

Absence of sensation in the abdomen, uterus, cervix and pelvic floor means the mother misses the usual feedback her body and pelvic floor gives during childbirth. Some mothers are able to sit up, others lie on their side with CTG, a drip in their arm and a catheter inserted to drain the bladder.

If an epidural is recommended and you are unsure, ask why it is being considered and remember your right to decline. For more information on epidurals: americanpregnancy.org/labornbirth/epidural.html, womenshealthmatters.ca/centres/pregnancy/childbirth/epidural.html

Episiotomy

Episiotomy is a full thickness cut through the perineal tissues to widen the vaginal opening as baby's head is crowning. It may be used during an emergency requiring immediate birth and should not be performed routinely. The use of episiotomy is an important issue to discuss with your birth atttendants prior to the birth.

Research shows there are few reasons to perform a routine episiotomy as it does not reduce the risk of tearing. A midline episiotomy, from the back of the vaginal opening towards the anus, cuts less muscle and is easier to repair, however it is more likely to extend into the anal sphincter. Extended tearing from an episiotomy (midline) is responsible for most 3rd and 4th degree tears. Tearing into the anal sphincter leads to faecal incontinence (poor control of wind and stool, and urgency). Early repair of this type of tear is paramount and is done soon after birthing. A mediolateral episiotomy, cutting down to the side at a 45–degree angle, involves more muscle damage in an attempt to reduce tearing.

Giving birth in supine (back-lying) increases the likelihood of having an episiotomy and perineal tearing. After the placenta is delivered the episiotomy incision is closed with dissolvable stitches.

Women who birth through an intact perineum are less likely to report vaginal pain during intercourse. Early management of scars following tearing or repair is discussed on page 110 and later stage scar mobilisation techniques on page 144. For more information on episiotomy: mayoclinic.com/health/episiotomy/HO00064

Birthing Position

The choice of birthing position has a significant impact on the outcome for baby and the pelvic floor. Studies of women (no epidural) found upright and left side-lying positions are associated with less pain during labour, lower use of episiotomy, vacumn extraction or forceps, fewer foetal heart abnormalities and a shorter pushing stage of labour.

Birthing by lying on the back or resting on the sacrum reduces the size of the pelvic outlet. The sacrum is prevented from slightly opening backwards to allow more space for baby's head. Lying on the back and raising the head to push during a contraction tightens the pelvic floor, which risks muscle tearing and/or an episiotomy. Different birthing positions will be encouraged by your midwife to shorten the second stage of labour and minimise pelvic floor trauma. Review different labour positions on page 72.

Other Interventions

Artificial rupture of the membranes (an induction or augmentation) breaks the watery membranes around baby. This procedure is used (often with a syntocinon drip), to start or speed up labour, to attach a monitor to baby's scalp or to check for meconium (baby poo) in the fluid. The soft cushioning membranes protect baby's soft skull from pressure during birth. When labour is prolonged or stops after membrane rupture, the risk of infection and time limits may prompt caregivers to intervene further. Many hospitals have time restrictions on birth and when labour slows or extends beyond 8 to 10 hours, further interventions are commenced.

A prolonged labour or slow to dilate cervix increases the risk of having the membranes broken, a drip inserted and being confined to bed by a monitor (avoided with telemetry). When the cervix is not sufficiently dilated, an induction may fail, resulting in birth by caesarean section.

Other methods to induce labour include placing prostaglandin gel on the cervix to cause softening and dilation. A small tube (Foley catheter) may be placed in the cervix with inflation of a small balloon to induce labour. To promote spontaneous labour, the birth attendant may insert a gloved finger through the cervix to 'stretch and sweep' the membranes.

Alternative methods of triggering labour include sexual intercourse (prostaglandins in semen can induce labour), nipple stimulation (oxytocin release can trigger labour), acupuncture, herbs and homeopathy (less research available on the risks and benefits).

Unless you have been advised otherwise, don't rush to hospital as soon as contractions start (despite what you see on television).

Labour proceeds more smoothly when the mother feels safe and relaxed, is free to move around without restriction, is well hydrated and supported by her birth partner and/or midwife. Becoming over-excited, fearful, stressed or anxious increases adrenalin levels causing labour to slow down or stop. Close the door, darken the room, stay off the bed, and focus on visualisation, breathing and pelvic rocking, to encourage contractions.

For more information on rupture of the membranes: midwife.org.nz/index.cfm/3,108,559/arm-consensus-statement-2008-final.pdf

Assisted vaginal birth involves the use of either forceps or a vacuum assisted suction (ventouse) to quickly birth baby during the second stage of labour. Forceps look like a pair of large salad tongs with a hole in the middle, which are shaped to fit around baby's head. During a contraction, the caregiver pulls as the mother pushes, to birth baby more quickly. They are used to turn the baby or for protection of a premature baby. With ventouse delivery, a cup is attached to baby's crown with a connective suction tube. The mother pushes during a contraction as the caregiver pulls to birth baby faster. Forceps or ventouse may be required when a 'heavy' epidural results in loss of leg movement or pelvic floor sensation.

Both forceps and vacuum extraction (to a lesser extent) cause higher rates of damage to the pelvic floor and internal supports. There is a greater risk of vaginal and perineal pain, bowel and urinary incontinence, and infection in stitches, following an assisted birth. When these procedures are performed without an episiotomy, the risk of deep perineal tearing is reduced. Some studies favour the use of vacuum assisted suction over forceps (when the birth attendant is a doctor), to reduce the risk of injury to the anal sphincter. Ask your doctor's preferred method if assistance is required for a quick birth.

Prolonged forceful pushing occurs when the mother is directed to bear down forcefully for long periods (with or without an epidural). This action can tear the vagina and pelvic floor, and strain internal supports. Spontaneous pushing is urge-driven by the mother; it is less tiring and reduces the risk of tearing. Pushing down on the mother's abdomen to help move the baby out is an unsafe practice and rarely used. In an emergency (where baby's shoulders are too wide for the pelvic outlet) this procedure may be used to rock baby's shoulder out from behind the pubic bone.

Following an instrument assisted birth, tearing or stitches, ask to see a women's health physiotherapist to ensure an effective pelvic floor recovery.

For more information on the risks and reasons for interventions, and your rights during childbirth: mybirth.com.au and childbirthconnection.org

Interventions and the Pelvic Floor

Key Points

- During pregnancy become informed about birthing practices used and their effect on the pelvic floor.
- Cardiotogram (CTG) limits a mother's ability to move around and is used to monitor baby's heartbeat when syntocinon is used.
- Epidural anaesthetic increases the risk of having an episiotomy, forceps delivery, vacuum extraction, or caesarean section.
- Episiotomy cuts through perineal muscles and should only be used during an emergency to quickly birth a baby who is not coping well.
- Lying on the back to birth risks more damage to the pelvic floor and increases the risk of having an episiotomy.
- Becoming over-excited, fearful, stressed or anxious increases adrenalin levels; labour may slow down or stop.
- Labour proceeds more smoothly when the mother feels safe and relaxed, is free to move around without restriction, and is well hydrated and supported by her birth partner and/or midwife.
- To encourage contractions: close the door, darken the room, stay off the bed, focus on visualization, breathing and pelvic rocking.
- Both forceps and vacuum extraction (to a lesser extent) have higher rates of damage to the pelvic floor and internal supports.
- Prolonged forceful pushing during labour for extended periods can injure the pelvic floor and internal supports.
- Spontaneous pushing is urge-driven by the mother; it is less tiring and reduces the risk of tearing.

Intervention questions to ask birth attendants:

SECTION 5

Birth

It is natural to be concerned about the effect of birth on PF muscle function. Pelvic floor outcomes are determined by many factors: interventions used, birthing positions, baby's position, size of the mother's pelvis, pain management choices, the choice of caregiver and birth setting. Some situations arise during labour requiring emergency intervention that clearly benefits the mother or baby, so discuss these situations beforehand.

Every woman has the right to know in advance the rate of interventions used at her birthing facility and the right to accept or refuse birthing practises. Ask birth attendants about their birthing practises and policies. To avoid practises known to cause problems, choose a birthing centre offering alternatives along with continuous support and care during labour.

Improving Pelvic Floor Outcomes

The following options may prevent or lessen pelvic floor damage, and conserve energy during labour.

Midwives are skilled professionals who provide support for the safest possible pregnancy, birth and postpartum recovery. Continuous care and help with decisions is provided over several months. Midwives are trained to understand and promote normal child bearing, use evidence-based interventions, and are skilled in managing emergency interventions. Research shows that fewer interventions are used when birthing is midwife led, it takes place in a quiet, calm birthing environment, and the mother's wishes are supported when possible.

Consider birthing with a **doula**, a non-midwife support person who is trained to offer support to the mother and her partner during birth and postpartum. Studies show midwives and doulas decrease the need for caesarean sections; requests for epidurals; length of labour for first time mothers; the use of narcotics; epidurals and forceps during labour.

Moving during labour, changing positions and walking helps baby move down into your pelvis. Movement shortens the first stage of labour and helps you respond to contractions in a positive way. Changing position moves the pelvic bones, allowing them to mould as baby finds the best fit to descend and rotate. Many women report changing positions speeds up labour after it slows. Researchers who found upright positions shortened the first stage of labour by 1 hour recommend that women should specifically be advised to avoid lying flat and to use upright positions they find comfortable during labour.

Lean forward onto pillows on the bed, kneel on hands and knees or circle your hips. When tired, sit on a ball or use a rocking chair to encourage rhythmic movement.

Hot towels and **hot packs** give comfort and pain relief when applied over the lower back and abdomen. Check if the hospital provides or permits you to bring hot packs. Use the **shower** to run warm water over your back for distraction, relaxation and pain relief while focusing on relaxed breathing to release muscle tension. Take a ball or stool into the shower to sit forwards with knees apart while the shower runs on your back. Use a hand held shower hose to direct water over your abdomen or back during contractions. Warm towels applied with pressure over the perineum during crowning are a comforting support to the pelvic floor as it stretches to release baby's head.

Water submersion promotes muscle relaxation and pain relief, supports body weight to gives a feeling of weightlessness and may shorten the length of labour. Special birthing tubs are bought or rented for home births. When birthing at a hospital, check if tubs are available, as not all hospitals accommodate water births. Women with high blood pressure, pre-eclampsia, diabetes or obesity are not suited to this type of birth. If heavy pain medication is used (beyond gas inhalation), or if baby is not coping well with labour, water submersion is avoided. Just as fingertips become soft and wrinkly after sitting in the bath, water helps perineal skin soften to minimise tearing.

In The Water Birth Book, Janet Balaskas recommends entering the birth tub or pool after labour is well established (5 to 6 centimeters dilated) as labour can slow down when a woman enters the tub too early. Many women have told me their most memorable births took place in the supporting comfort of warm water either in an outdoor hot tub or in a quiet, darkened room with soft music.

Massage is a great pain reliever, providing comfort and confidence during labour. Thumb kneading down the neck and across the shoulders, and firm stroking down the spine relieves muscle tension. Partner thumb pressure over the skin dimples of the sacrum counters the intensity of 'back labour' pain. Firm, slow, deep pressure is important, as a light or nervous touch is often annoying. Encourage your partner to try these techniques during pregnancy as preparation for labour. Most likely you will know exactly the area you want massaged and direct partners when to start and stop, although some women who normally love massage find it annoying or unpleasant at times.

Warn partners the pressure required may fatigue their hands. Tell them to get over it and help you out. A massage tool or oil makes it easier to provide deeper pressure and reduces tiring of the hands. During crowning and following birth, midwives sometimes massage frozen fingers of ice over the perineum to reduce perineal swelling and bruising.

One study compared the effect of **music** on pain in a group of labouring women, with women who laboured without music. The study involved first time mothers listening to calming music, with measurements of pain perception and intensity done hourly after 3–4 centimeters dilation. The music group reported less pain and emotional distress, leading the researchers to promote calming music as 'an effective, easy to use alternative to pain medication, for easing pain during early labour'.

TENS (transcutaneous electrical nerve stimulation) is used during labour to block pain messages to the brain and release natural painkillers (endorphins). Small adhesive electrodes are placed over nerve points on the low back and buttocks and attached to a small, hand-held battery-operated device. The intensity is adjusted to a lower frequency to stimulate endorphin release or a higher frequency to ease pain. To stimulate labour contractions, the electrodes are placed over acupressure points. TENS is most effective when used from early labour and cannot be used with water.

Compression stockings are worn *during labour* to support leg veins when pregnancy has caused varicose veins. The graded garment pressure counteracts dilation and pressure on leg veins during labour to prevent further varicosities.

Acupuncture is used over specific body points to raise or lower energy levels before labour starts. Needling helps to stimulate uterine contractions after the amniotic sac has broken and contractions have stopped, or when pregnancy goes over 40 weeks. When administered by an experienced, registered acupuncturist, it is an effective, non-invasive method to induce contractions, ease the intensity of contractions and shorten labour time.

Aromatherapy is used with massage or by burning certain oils to help stimulate contractions. As naked flames (candles) are not permitted in hospitals, choose an electric burner. Aroma therapists commonly use the following oils—clary sage (not recommended with epilepsy), jasmine, lavender, chamomile, mandarin, geranium or rose.

Positioning for Labour

As labour progresses, it is normal to rotate through different positions as baby moves out of the uterus into the pelvis for birth. Changing positions (combined with pelvic movement, massage, water, dim lights, music, distraction techniques, focused breathing and emotional support) is part of effective pain management in labour. Adopt comfortable upright positions as uterine contractions move baby down to the pelvic floor. Lying on the back slows labour and increases the risk of interventions. Imagine how ineffective and difficult bowel emptying would also become in this position. Stay active and find comfortable positions to labour and rest between contractions. Practise some of these different positions with your partner.

- Slow dancing from foot to foot while leaning into your partner (take a digital player loaded with your favourite calming music).
- Squatting encourages faster descent into the pelvis—try partial squatting with buttocks pushed out behind and forearms resting on the bed.
- Sit on the ball if you are tired from standing or squatting. Ball sitting supports thighs and takes pressure off the perineum while keeping the pressure of baby's head down onto the cervix. Try using the ball in the shower.
- Sit on the ball or birthing stool with knees wide apart to open the pelvic floor and hips. Lean forward and rest forearms on thighs. When pushing, use the same opening action as when your bowel opens (page 25).
- Straddle a kitchen chair (no arms), leaning on the chair back and

keeping the spine straight to avoid slumping.

- Sit your birth partner on a ball pushed against the wall. With back to your partner, squat in front of the ball while they support under your armpits. Rest your arms on their thighs. Use this same position for birthing in the tub (without ball).

- Try a 'hanging' squat position with a towel wrapped over a *strong* rail; hold onto the ends of the towel with both hands and go down into a squat.

- To help ease pain during 'back labour', kneel on a pillow and rest forearms on the ball or wrap arms around it, rocking gently back and forth to ease back pain. This is an ideal position for your partner to give back massage and apply heat packs.

- Sterile water injections under the skin overlying the sacrum brings effective relief of 'back labour' pain in 60 per cent of women, with the effect lasting up to 2 hours.

- When baby is descending at an angle, some midwives advise lunging to encourage turning the baby. Face a chair placed against the wall. Put one foot on the chair and lunge forward into the chair. Repeat several times before changing legs.

- Keep pressure off the sacrum and coccyx by avoiding a back-lying or supported back-lying position, which prevents the sacral joints from slightly opening to create more space for baby.

- To slow a fast labour, recover some energy or when intervention (epidural) is required, move to left side lying. Your partner can help by supporting your upper leg to open the pelvis if you birth in this position.

- *When birth takes place in a tub, raise body weight off the buttocks, kneel or squat with one knee on the floor of the tub and the other foot flat.*

Progressing Through Labour

Use simple breathing skills during labour to keep you (and baby) well oxygenated, more relaxed and to conserve energy. Focused breathing helps you use contractions to progress labour rather than tightening up and slowing progress.

Learn breathing skills before labour to avoid breath holding and build confidence in managing contractions. Practice the focused breathing contained in this section while sitting in a favourite chair, in the bath, under the shower, while pelvic circling, or kneeling on hands and knees.

If you experience Braxton Hicks uterine contractions in later pregnancy, this is a perfect time to stop and focus or breathing and visualization. The uterine muscles contract for 30 to 60 seconds but occasionally this type of contraction lasts for up to 2 minutes. Braxton Hicks contractions may have the effect of softening the cervix during later pregnancy.

Involve your birth partner so they know how to coach and refocus breath control at different stages throughout labour. Try breathing together with full eye contact and following your partner's breathing pattern to recover focus if you become over-whelmed during a contraction. Closing the eyes during contractions is normal.

Before labour, choose a 'touch code' so your partner can help you settle during any anxious moments, e.g. your partner places a hand on your shoulder as the signal for you to breathe out slowly.

Prenatal yoga and meditation develop relaxation skills and focused breathing techniques in different positions. These lifetime skills can be used during any stressful life crises.

Stage 1: Early Labour (cervix dilates 0–3 cms)

Early labour contractions soften, shorten and begin to open the cervix. Hours or days before contractions begin, the mucus 'plug' (show) in the cervix sometimes comes out and this 'show' is a sign labour is not too far away. When it is released in early labour you may not even notice it has happened.

Mild period-like cramps or dull backache signal labour is probably not far away. As the cervix dilates, healthy uterine contractions become increasingly regular and stronger during this early stage of labour.

The early contractions are shorter (15 to 40 seconds), irregular in pattern and usually more than five minutes apart. Listen to your body, sleep or take a bath to become more comfortable. The sac of amniotic fluid can break at any time—either before contractions begin or more commonly they break later in labour, shortly before or during the pushing stage. Some women find their labour starts then stops, while for others, it progresses smoothly.

Breathe in deeply at the start of a contraction and blow out slowly through pursed lips, keeping your jaw relaxed. Avoid breath holding.

First babies often take their time and women who have already given birth usually find their labour is shorter. There is no way to predict the length of labour. Rest and eat lighter foods (yoghurt and fruit are easily digested) to avoid overloading the stomach, and vomiting. Keep hydrated with water and juices.

Unless otherwise advised, stay at home until labour is well established before entering hospital.

Stage 1: Active Labour (cervix dilates 3–7 cm)

The sac of amniotic fluid protects baby during contractions and often does not break until active labour. Contractions now become longer, stronger and more frequent as the cervix continues to open. It's normal to feel period type ache or low back discomfort as the cervix dilates. Now is the time to use visualization skills as contractions arrive more frequently than in early labour. They start slowly and build up to a stronger peak before fading away and are typically 3 to 5 minutes apart, lasting from 45 to 90 seconds until the cervix is fully dilated.

Adopt forward and upright positions to maximize optimal foetal positioning for birth. Try different positions to find the most comfortable and rest between contractions to conserve energy. Movement, belly dancing, hip circling on a ball, massage, a bath or shower are helpful. Water immersion in a bath is used when labour is well advanced and if there are no complications and maternal BMI is below 35. The immersion provides comfort through support and a feeling of weightlessness.

Transition Stage (cervix dilates 7–10 cm)

During this later stage of labour, the cervix opens up to 10 centimetres, for entry of baby's head into the vagina. Muscles at the top of the uterus contract to push baby's head down onto the cervix to help with further dilation. Contractions are stronger, lasting for 60 to 90 seconds and are 1 to 3 minutes apart during this stage, which lasts from 30 minutes to 2 hours. The transition stage is brief for some women and for others, a challenging time with temporary shaking, nausea, impatience, and a strong desire to open the bowel.

Partners may also feel overwhelmed and often look to the midwife for reassurance. It helps partners to know this is all part of a normal process and what you are experiencing is 'healthy' birth pain, not damaging pain.

This is the time for partners to step up into the coaching role (using your 'touch code') through this often-intense stage, even when told, in no uncertain terms, where to go! Partner coaching involves giving massage, encouraging you to rock or circle the hips, bringing cool face cloths, offering sips of fluid, helping with position changes, providing verbal encouragement and reminders to breathe while keeping eye-to-eye contact, until this shorter, intense stage passes. Sometimes partners need to be quiet and appreciate you may not want to be touched.

If labour slows down during this stage, start moving with hip rocking, or get into a warm tub or shower, which may reduce the need for drugs to intensify labour. Try sitting on a birth stool or the toilet to relax and open the pelvic floor. Your birth attendant may suggest breaking the membranes, which usually brings on stronger contractions.

If labour does not progress (dilation of cervix slower than 1 cm per hour), an intravenous drip containing the artificial version of oxytocin or syntocinon (the labour hormone) may be used to encourage or promote contractions. As the hormone drip brings on strong, frequent contractions, you will need to be creative and have more support to cope with the artificially strong contractions. If the syntocinon drip is well managed, the contractions should not be overwhelming. Enquire beforehand about your caregivers or hospitals policy on speeding up a slow labour.

When syntocinon is used, baby's heartbeat is regularly monitored for signs they are not coping, by a cardiotocograph (CTG) machine (refer to monitoring on page 60).

Use the focused breathing below with the start of each contraction.

- Take a deep in-breath and breathe out a long 'har' sound through an opened mouth, and focus on making a low vibration sensation in the base of your throat. Repeat the 'throat sound' breathing throughout the contraction.

- Practise making the low throat sounds softly, then more loudly on the out-breath with a relaxed, open jaw *and* pelvic floor. High or shrill noises tighten the PF muscles.
- Focusing on the low back of throat vibrations during the out breath avoids breath holding or hyperventilating (rapid upper chest breathing).
- Use the breathing with throat sounds and visualise the cervix opening to a 10 centimeters wide circle.
- In the last weeks of pregnancy practise this visualisation with a cut out 10cm wide circle with 2, 4, 6 and 8 centimetre inner circles. Use the circle during labour to focus on opening the cervix during contractions. Birthing involves creating an opening for baby rather than pushing as hard as possible.

Sometimes there is an overwhelming desire to push even when the midwife tells you not to push until the cervix is fully dilated. Try getting into the 'head down-bum up' position and start quicker 'har' vocalised breathing on the out-breath to prevent early pushing. Lying on your side may also help to overcome an early urge to push.

Stage 2: Full dilation of cervix to birth of baby

After full cervix dilation, the uterus and vagina are continuous, allowing baby to leave the uterus and descend to the pelvic floor. A resting phase of up to 20 minutes is normal as the uterus prepares for active pushing. Research on the effect of pushing on the birth outcome showed the women who pushed immediately after full dilation, recorded higher caesarean and instrument assisted birth rates. The researchers advised women to delay pushing until a reflexive urge to do so, which also significantly reduced the mothers postpartum fatigue.

When baby descends with spontaneous pushing, the pelvic and perineal tissues adjust to the strain, thereby reducing vaginal and perineal trauma.

If you have not recently emptied your bladder, do so now to prevent obstruction to baby's head. Bowel emptying between contractions is common, as the bowel muscles contract along with the uterus. Don't push until you feel an urge to do so and choose a comfortable gravity assisted position. Lie on your side if you are feeling exhausted. This stage is usually faster for women who have previously given birth and from 1 to 2 hours for first time mothers.

Stage 3: Crowning and birth of baby

This stage typically lasts from 5 to 15 minutes. During crowning, your body usually pushes instinctively. When baby makes contact with the pelvic floor, the involuntary urge to push is compelling and this effort, combined with uterine contractions, guides baby through the pelvic floor.

Breathing out with throat sounds and a relaxed jaw assists internal bearing down using your diaphragm; a through body muscle which attaches to the ribs and lower sternum in front, and the mid to lower spine at the back. Juju Sundin compares the action of using the diaphragm to bear down onto the uterus, to a coffee plunger pushing down. For dizziness or light-headedness, cup both hands over your mouth and breathe back carbon dioxide to relieve the sensations.

When baby's head crowns, a stretching, stinging or burning sensation is felt, although this varies between women. The midwife may ask you to stop pushing for a while to slow down the birth and let your perineum stretch more slowly. Applying hot face cloths to the vaginal, perineal and anal area gives wonderful relief at this point. Supporting the perineal and anal areas with warm towel pressure is useful to help prevent tearing. If the perineum is swollen, ice massage may be used to reduce swelling and postpartum bruising.

When an epidural is performed, little sensation or feedback is felt from the pelvic floor. In this case a mirror can be used so the mother sees her pelvic floor with midwife finger pressure showing her where to push. Stretching the pelvic floor open (as with perineal massage) is avoided during crowning as it aggravates swelling, bruising and tearing.

To assist the pelvic floor:

- Move to standing, kneeling on all fours or kneeling with one foot flat on the floor, for gravity assisted descent of baby into the pelvis and through the pelvic floor. Lying in the left lateral position to birth is also associated with less perineal damage.
- A strong pressure sensation on the rectum is felt as baby's head descends. It's not unusual to lose wind or small amounts of bowel contents.
- To push during a contraction, use the same releasing action as when your bowel opens. *Practise this action by placing both hands either side of your waist. Make a long, low 'har' sound (this widens the waist) and open your pelvic floor.*
- This pushing action uses the diaphragm and transversus abdominis, protecting the rectus abdominis from further strain during the pushing stage of labour.
- The perineum bulges as baby's head crowns and stretches the PF muscles and vulva, with the top and back of the head visible (the scalp looks crinkly but smooths out later). In the normal birthing situation, baby's back is under the abdomen and their face is towards the mother's spine.
- Baby's head starts to turn after it makes contact with the pelvic floor. The chin tucks down so the crown of the head presents and is birthed first, then the head extends to release the chin.
- When directed to stop pushing as baby's head crowns, resume the short open-mouthed 'har' throat sounds, then *slowly* birth

baby's head to prevent tearing.

- Using a mirror lets you see the crown and progress made. Don't be discouraged if part of baby's head emerges then slips back vaginally, because passage of the head is close; it's normal for baby's head to move back slightly after each contraction. Some midwives cup or support the vulva as baby's head advances into the world.

- *Assist the pelvic floor by gently placing your hand on baby's head and slowly 'breathing' baby out into your hand.*

- Once baby's head is fully exposed, it turns towards one of your legs to allow the shoulders and body to slip out.

Other Presentations

A *breech* presentation is where baby's bottom half presents first into the birth canal as opposed to the head. During late pregnancy, external manipulation and massage may be used to turn baby into the head down (vertex) position. Breech vaginal birth is not advised for first time mothers.

Some babies present *posteriorly* with their back against the mother's spine or towards the mother's left or right side instead of anteriorly. While the majority turn to the front during labour, others remain in the posterior or rotated position. These presentations slow birth, particularly for first time mothers, with pressure of baby's head on the sacrum.

At routine checkups ask which way baby is positioned. External manipulation can start at 34 weeks to decrease the likelihood of baby being in the posterior position when labour commences. When the birth attendant uses internal head rotation during labour, this manoeuvre should not be attempted until the cervix is fully dilated (to avoid injury to the cervix).

The following strategies may encourage a baby to turn from a posterior to an anterior presentation:

- Before labour, regularly kneel or crawl on hands and knees on the carpet for 5–10 minutes.
- Swim or use a kick board in the pool.
- March on the spot or step up and down on a stair with handrail support.
- Move into the 'head down, bottom up' position during labour, to tip baby out of the pelvis so there is more space for baby to turn.
- Kneel on hands and knees with hip circling and rocking to ease back pain.
- Apply regular heat packs, showers and deep massage (with oil) for lower back pain.
- Avoid lying on your back or deep squatting, which reduces the space for baby to turn.
- Sit on the birth chair or toilet in a forward leaning position.
- Lie on your side when tired.

Stage 4: Placental delivery and early postpartum care

After baby is born, uterine contractions and the urge to push resumes to separate the placenta from the uterine wall. In hospital, syntocinon is routinely injected into the thigh to speed up placental separation, decrease bleeding and the risk of hemorrhage. This stage takes from five to 20 minutes and is substantially longer without the injection.

Physiological third stage, without injection (natural placental delivery) may take between 1 to 3 hours. It avoids syntocinon injection and the risk of placental tearing caused through pulling the placenta from the uterus. Studies shows that natural placental delivery is safe for women at low risk of postpatum haemorrhage and that 'active management' is associated with a seven to eight fold increase in postpartum haemorrhage for women in the study groups. Delaying cord cutting allows baby to receive all the cord blood and clotting factors, while attaching to the breast or staying on their mother's chest (with a warm blanket cover).

Holding your baby in a warm peaceful environment and breastfeeding as soon as possible, stimulates uterine contractions to expel the placenta and stop bleeding at the site where the placenta detaches from the uterus.

The placenta and membranes are examined to ensure that all has separated and come away. Syntocinon is sometimes used to stimulate contractions to assist placental detachment (with active management). However it is less effective when it was used earlier to speed up the birth.

Caesarean Birth

An elective caesarean is scheduled before labour commences and an emergency caesarean is performed during labour, due to a medical emergency. When labour is not progressing, the birth needs to happen quickly or the risk to mother and baby is thought to be too great with a vaginal birth, a caesarean birth is preferred. Epidurals and spinal anaesthetic are most commonly used to perform a caesarean, with general anaesthetic used when a medical emergency occurs, the epidural is not working effectively or the mother prefers this type of anaesthetic.

Debate continues to surround the increasing rate of caesarean births, as some caregivers prefer this mode of birth and some women view it as a birth option when there is no medical indication for its use. The World Health Organization (WHO) has a long-term goal of reducing the caesarean rate and recommends a rate of 10 to 15 per cent. The present rate in Australia is around 30 per cent (in 1977 the rate was 10 per cent). Some private hospitals have caesarean rates close to 60 per cent. While a caesarean section prevents (occasional) major PF muscle damage, it does not provide protection against bladder incontinence and prolapse in the longer term.

Following a caesarean birth, the majority of women have a repeat caesarean for subsequent births. Women who wish to birth vaginally after a prior caesarean (VBAC) require more support and often feel isolated when their family and caregiver do not support their decision.

During a surgical birth, a 15 to 20 centimetre horizontal, low caesarean incision (low bikini line) cuts through skin and fat, then the abdominal muscles, and fascial layers. The peritoneum (sac lining the abdomen and pelvis and covering the abdominal contents) is retracted down to the bladder, which sits in front of the uterus. The bladder is moved down and a 10 to 12 centimetre horizontal cut is made into the lower area of the uterus.

One of three different types of incisions will be used during a caesarean:

- A transverse or horizontal incision into the lower part of the uterus. This incision (which is most commonly used) heals with less scarring and a much lower chance of rupturing with future pregnancy.

- A vertical incision cuts from the middle to the upper section of the uterus (and is only rarely used) to birth baby quickly, during a medical emergency.

- A low vertical incision cuts into the lower section of the uterus (and is only rarely used) if the surgeon is uncertain whether an upper vertical incision is necessary.

The surgeon lifts baby up and out of the uterus and removes the placenta from the uterine wall. The uterus is closed with two (sometimes one) layers of dissolving stitches followed by the linea alba (band into which all abdominal muscles attach). The peritoneum is commonly left open and not resutured.

Longer-term studies are required to evaluate future outcomes for adhesions, subsequent pregnancies and births with peritoneal closure and non-closure. The skin is closed with a further layer of dissolving, removable or occasionally, metal staples. A small plastic drain may be temporarily left in place to remove excess blood.

Birth

Key Points

- Assist labour by engaging a midwife (and doula), using tens, acupuncture and aromatherapy.
- Effective pain management in labour involves changing positions, pelvic movement, massage, water, dim lights, calming music, distraction techniques, focused breathing and emotional support.
- Adopt comfortable upright positions as uterine contractions move baby down to the pelvic floor. Lying on the back slows labour and increases the risk of interventions.
- Before labour, choose a 'touch code' so your partner can help you settle during any anxious moments.
- Use relaxed jaw breathing with low throat sounds and visualise the cervix opening to a 10 centimeters wide circle.
- If labour slows down during the active stage, start moving with hip rocking, or get into a warm tub or shower, which may reduce the need for drugs to intensify labour.
- Pushing before baby's head reaches the pelvic floor, risks damage to the vagina. Try getting into the 'head down-bum up' position and start quicker 'har' vocalised breathing on the out-breath to prevent early pushing.
- Supporting the perineal and anal areas with warm towel pressure during crowning helps to prevent tearing.
- Ask for baby to be immediately placed on your chest and covered with a warm blanket as contact and breast feeding encourages uterine contractions and hormone production.

Birth questions to ask birth attendants:

SECTION 6

Early PostPartum

Birth is a life transition with great potential for growth and transformation, bringing all sorts of changes and challenges. New motherhood is a mixture of excitement and sleep deprivation; of joy and exhaustion. It's all too easy to overlook your need to restore optimal strength and functional stability to meet the physical and emotional demands of parenting.

Postpartum is an important time to protect, heal and re-strengthen the pelvic floor and abdominal muscles, as these muscles are central to restoring abdominal and trunk muscle length and synergistic function.

This section contains advice on common postpartum pelvic issues regardless of the mode of birth, followed by different sections for vaginal and caesarean mothers. It presents ways to recover strength and avoid further pelvic floor and physical ailments while settling into your role as a new mother. I have included a questionnaire for recording specific issues that are sometimes overlooked in the busy postpartum period. Show the results to caregivers for appropriate advice, treatment, or referral as early treatment lowers the risk of future dysfunction.

Fill out the self-reporting questionnaire before leaving hospital (2–7 days after birth), and again at 6 weeks, 6 months and 12 months postpartum.

Seek treatment for altered bladder or bowel control, pain, or signs of prolapse, and keep a track of changes over the next 12 months. This chart allows you to assess whether the symptoms are improving and to look at different treatment options if progress has stalled.

Scoring is on a scale of one to ten, where one is minimal pain or level of bother, and ten is severe pain or level of bother.

New Mother Pelvic Floor Questionnaire

	Week 1	Week 6	Month 6	Month 12
Urine loss with exertion				
Urine loss with urgency				
Poor wind or stool control or bowel urgency				
Hemorrhoids, constipation, pain on emptying, fissures				
Pain in back, pelvis, groin or abdomen				
Infected scars, stitches				
Vaginal 'falling out' feeling				
Sexual pain				
Scar pain				
Diastasis Rectus				

Diastasis Rectus Abdominis

Diastasis rectus abdominis (DRA) is common due to extreme abdominal wall stretching during pregnancy. The diastasis improves in the majority of women with wearing abdominal muscle supports, avoiding forward trunk curling movements and an ongoing commitment to strengthening transversus abdominis (with the pelvic floor). In those affected 53 per cent are separated immediately postpartum and 36 per cent remain abnormally wide at 5 to 7 weeks postpartum.

A diastasis looks like an abdominal midline domed bulge when the head is bent forwards from a back lying position. Some women develop a golf ball sized 'pop out' at their belly button, which indicates an umbilical hernia. When a separation of 2.7 centimeters or more lasts longer than 4 weeks, research associates this gap with persistent lower back, pubic symphysis and sacroiliac joint pain and incontinence. A persistent gap prevents the abdominals from generating enough force to stabilise the pelvis and spine during activity.

To test for or measure the diastasis:

- Lie on your back with both knees bent.
- Place middle fingers of one hand over the belly button with fingers pointing down towards your toes.
- Lift your head forwards and feel the firm ridges of the rectus muscle either side of your fingers. As you feel the sides of the muscle coming together, note the number of fingers that fit down into the gap. Wait 6 to 8 weeks after a caesarean before doing this test.

The following actions will promote healing of the strained abdominal connective tissues.

- Immediately postpartum wear a cross over diastasis splint with velcro closure or the long line recovery shorts. I have seen good closure in women wearing both garments. Wear these supports 24/7 to keep the muscle bellies closer together as the underlying abdominal connective tissues heal.
- Wearing these supports is not enough. Forward trunk curling

movements or exercises must always be avoided as this action pulls the rectus bellies apart.

- Combined with a splint or shorts, consistent strengthening of the transversus abdominis muscle is the most effective way to close the diastasis. Use pelvic floor lifting to switch on transversus.
- Start the Jellybelly exercises on page 155 and focus on breathing, postural control, lifting only baby and strengthening the transversus with the pelvic floor. Transversus is the muscle responsible for flattening the abdomen.
- Progress to the 'Hissy lift' (page 159) initially in sitting for 2 to 4 weeks then repeat the action in standing (wearing support).
- Roll onto your side to get out of bed and prevent the trunk curling action.
- Prior to being fitted with a splint or shorts, add abdominal hand support to protect your abdomen. Cross both arms over your abdomen with one hand on either side of the separated muscle. Pull the hands and muscles towards the navel with coughing or forward body movements.
- Avoid carrying baby in a low sling or back carrier until the diastasis is closed. Keep baby high and close to your chest.
- Avoid lifting and twisting actions e.g. placing a toddler in a car seat. Move the feet to keep hips and shoulders facing in the same direction. Re-read specific exercises to avoid on page 32.

The wider the gap, the longer the rehabilitation of your abdominal wall will take. When the rectus muscles (and underlying connective tissues) do not regain sufficient closure by 12 months postpartum, surgical repair with a plastic surgeon may be necessary to improve function. Prior to surgery diagnostic ultrasound is used to assess the extent of connective tissue damage before deciding to proceed with the repair.

Successful repair is underpinned by prior retraining of transversus to ensure the abdominals work in a coordinated manner. Post surgically a well functioning transversus prevents the stitches being strained and lowers the risk of a future diastasis.

Bladder Control

Temporary loss of bladder control after vaginal and caesarean birth responds well to committed PF exercises. The most common type of postpartum urine loss is leaking during sneezing, lifting or exercise, when exertion increases intra-abdominal pressure. Research results indicate that stress incontinence following the first birth is a significant indicator of stress incontinence 12 years later.

Urge loss occurs when bladder muscles spasm. Control sudden bladder urgency by tightening the PC muscle, curling toes under and breathing until the urge passes. Ideally, the bladder should empty five or six times a day and once at night (depending on fluid intake), so persist with bladder training to delay emptying until you can hold at least 250 to 300mls before voiding. Months or years after birth, urgency can be related to untreated scar adhesions and muscular trigger points.

If normal bladder signals are absent or urine does not release following birth, inform your caregiver immediately as a temporary urinary catheter is required to drain the bladder and prevent over distension. Urine flow is often heavier in the early postpartum days as the body eliminates excess pregnancy fluids.

Sitting on the toilet and relaxing the pelvic floor normally triggers bladder muscle contraction (bladder muscles are not under voluntary control). Toileting with abdominal tension prevents complete PF muscle relaxation and leads to the habit of pushing down to pass urine, which is one cause of bladder urgency. *Develop a healthy lifetime habit of voiding with abdominal wall relaxation in a tall sitting posture.*

Weaker bladder control postpartum is effectively controlled with regular PF exercises. Around 24 to 48 hours following an uncomplicated vaginal birth, start gentle PF exercises. Review the *Shrink the jellybelly* program on page 155. When a catheter is inserted to drain urine, begin PF exercises after the catheter is removed.

Even with good postpartum bladder control, add exercises to your daily health routine to ensure the pelvic floor copes with the demands of activity and lifting growing children, along with preventing incontinence and prolapse at menopause when hormonal changes lead to weakening of urethral control. Women who practise regular PF exercises are more likely to retain strength of this muscle group into senior years.

When bladder (or bowel) weakness persists after returning home, despite diligently repeating PF exercises, fill out the bladder (or bowel) charts starting page 184, and show the completed form to your caregivers as incontinence rarely goes away by itself. Following a healthy eating plan, combined with regular PF exercises, is essential to control postpartum and future incontinence. **Researchers have identified less incontinence at 6 months postpartum in mothers who had lost pregnancy weight gains.**

Prolapse

Pelvic organs herniate or slip down into the vaginal walls when pelvic supports stretch and PF muscles fail to close and lift. Prolapse occurs in 50 per cent of childbearing women and those with few symptoms may be unaware of this condition until a bulge presents at the vaginal entrance. Prolapse can affect one or more pelvic organs: the symptoms associated with specific prolapses are listed below.

The **vaginal anterior or front wall prolapse** occurs when the bladder or urethra descends into the front vaginal wall (Fig.7). Commonly reported symptoms are:

- urine loss with coughing and activity
- bulging at the front of the vaginal entrance with coughing
- tampons fall out
- bladder emptying problems
- incomplete emptying, recurrent bladder infections
- discomfort or pain during intercourse

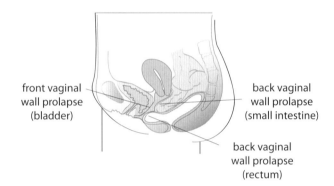

front vaginal wall prolapse (bladder)

back vaginal wall prolapse (small intestine)

back vaginal wall prolapse (rectum)

Fig. 7. Front and back vaginal wall prolapse

The **vaginal posterior or back wall prolapse** occurs when the **rectum** descends into the back vaginal wall (Fig. 7) with the following symptoms:

- difficult and/or incomplete bowel emptying requiring digital help
- straining to empty
- bulging at the back of the vaginal entrance with coughing
- difficult to retain a tampon
- discomfort or pain with intercourse

When the **small intestine** descends into the upper back vaginal wall between the uterus and rectum (Fig. 7), common symptoms are:

- constipation and difficult bowel emptying

- rectal pressure sensation
- lower back pain worse after prolonged standing
- vaginal discharge or bleeding
- discomfort or pain with intercourse

Utero-vaginal descent occurs when the cervix (and uterus) descends vaginally (Fig. 8). Women with a retroverted uterus (the uterus tips backwards towards the spine in 20 per cent of women) are more at risk of developing an advanced stage of this type of prolapse and requiring surgical correction.

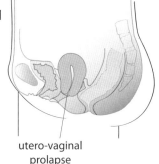

utero-vaginal
prolapse

Fig. 8. Utero-vaginal prolapse

Symptoms include:

- urinary incontinence
- constipation
- low back pain
- vaginal and pelvic heaviness
- menstrual type cramps
- painful intercourse

Vaginal vault prolapse affects women who have previously had a hysterectomy. The upper part of the vagina sags down into the lower vagina and common symptoms are:

- vaginal pressure
- painful intercourse
- back pain
- urinary incontinence

Rectal prolapse occurs when the rectum descends through the anus due to nerve damage with chronic bowel straining, diarrhea or multiple sclerosis, and is more common with advancing age. Another form of prolapsed rectum is called internal intussusception, where the upper rectum slides down inside the rectum like a tube within a tube.

Risk of prolapse

White and Latina women have the highest rate of prolapse followed by Asian and African-American women. If your mother had a prolapse your risk increases by threefold. There is an increased risk around menopause for women with several children and a larger waist measurement. Large uterine fibroids, pelvic tumors and excessive abdominal weight place more internal pressure down onto pelvic organs, requiring more effort from the PF muscles to counter the internal pressure. Chronic bowel straining, coughing with chest disease, heavy lifting and over challenging exercise set the scene for prolapse. When pushing occurs before the reflexive urge, the second stage of labour is prolonged, forceps or suction is required, and the first time mother is over 35, the risk of prolapse is increased.

Prolapse will not go away by itself, however not all cases of prolapse require surgery. An internal exam determines the type of prolapse and sometimes a referral for an ultrasound or magnetic resonance imaging test is needed to determine the degree of prolapse (refer to self-examination for prolapse starting on page 128).

Women with a mild to moderate degree of prolapse find their prolapse responds positively to lifestyle changes and PF muscle strengthening. Fitting a pessary support to reposition the prolapsed organ(s) makes it easier to lift and strengthen PF muscles.

Pessaries

The pessary support is a ring shaped device (shapes vary) inserted high vaginally to reduce and relieve prolapse symptoms and prevent the prolapse from worsening. Many different types are available and your caregiver will select and fit the most appropriate pessary for the type of prolapse. Fitting is by trial and error and it's not unusual to change the size or type a few days or months later. When a pessary falls out, it is either too small or too large or the vagina is open or too short.

Surgeons sometimes insert a pessary to relieve symptoms while waiting for surgery, or if surgery is not possible due to existing medical conditions. Pessary management includes returning every 3 months for removal, cleaning, vaginal wall inspection and refitting. Some women prefer to remove the pessary at night and reinsert in the morning. They are used in younger women to relieve bladder incontinence, support an incompetent pregnant cervix and reduce a prolapse after childbirth. Menopausal women use oestrogen cream with the pessary to improve the quality of vaginal tissues.

Practical front line strategies to prevent pelvic organ descent are avoiding the causes, improving posture, changing damaging habits and making PF exercise a part of everyday health routines.

Suggested actions:

- Ask your doctor or enquire at a women's clinic about fitting a vaginal pessary to lift and support internal organs and continue working on PF strength exercises.
- Sit, stand and walk tall by lengthening through the crown of your head to keep PF and abdominal core muscles active.
- Practise the 'knack' (page 21) by lifting PF muscles before picking up children and baby capsules, coughing or sneezing.
- Avoid lifting more than baby until PF and core muscles are stronger.
- *Bowel straining causes postpartum prolapse. Use a pad to support your perineum as the bowel opens. Eat fibre-rich food and drink more water to keep stools soft. Use a fibre rich emulsion such as fibogel or metamucil to soften stools.*
- Treat a chest infection or allergic sneezing early.

- Avoid pushing yourself during exercise classes as PF muscles may fail under the load of challenging or prolonged exercise.
- Return to easy exercise such as regular walking and swimming in the first four to six months to strengthen the abdomen and trunk.
- Consider learning slow belly dancing (or latin dance) to develop control and strength in pelvic and abdominal muscles.

Pelvic Girdle Pain (PGP)

For most women, PGP disappears by 12 weeks postpartum, however pain persists in 10 per cent for 1 to 2 years. Those with pubic symphysis, sacroiliac joint and hip pain have a slower rate of recovery when compared to women with fewer sites of pain. When PGP continues there is an increased risk of chronic lumbopelvic pain later in life, making early treatment of this condition a high priority.

Wearing a support garment is like adding an extra protective layer of muscles to protect joints, support muscles, reposition organs, reduce swelling and encourage correct posture immediately postpartum. Stabilising exercises for the pelvic floor and core muscles (starting with the Find It, Train It program on page 163) are a main focus of postpartum exercise for women with PGP. Always seek assessment of any persistent pain to gain accurate diagnosis and treatment.

Under-activity of the thyroid gland or a flare up of pre-existing rheumatoid arthritis (that improves during pregnancy) may now aggravate joint pain. For further information on PGP: pelvicinstability.org.au or pelvicpartnership.org.uk

Back Pain

The way women use their trunk and pelvic muscles changes during pregnancy and correcting altered postural and movement patterns are integral to preventing ongoing dysfunction. Postpartum is a crucial time to learn dynamic stability so all the pelvic and trunk muscles work in a synergistic or balanced pattern. If stability is not restored, faulty patterns of movement cause ongoing pelvic weakness with longer-term back and PGP, diastasis rectus, prolapse and incontinence.

Some women develop back pain following the effort of labour or due to the dramatic change in their centre of gravity and body shape. Suddenly, ligaments, joints and muscles are working in a different posture. Back pain in the early postpartum period is also related to poor posture, spending long periods in a trunk flexed position to breastfeed, pelvic organ prolapse and picking up older children, and is associated with poor function in pelvic floor, core and trunk muscles.

Try this quick test of pelvic floor and core muscle coordination:

Lie on your back with legs straight and lift one leg a few inches off the floor. If the abdomen bulges upwards and the pelvic floor descends, the core muscles are not tightening to stabilise the pelvis. The curve in the lower back should not flatten during this test. Normally, in response to leg lifting, the abdomen firms and flattens in conjunction with pelvic floor lifting, Difficulty lifting one leg (compared to the other leg lift), indicates specific pelvic floor muscle or sacroiliac joint problems.

Restore dynamic control by maintaining tall postures and continuing with a program of pelvic floor and core rehabilitation.

Ease spinal aches and pains with the following actions:

- Sit, stand and walk tall to keep PF and core postural muscles continually active.

- As soon as possible, start the PF and core exercise program.
- Review the coughing test on page 23, to ensure your pelvic floor is lifting and coordinating with other abdominal muscles.
- Wear an elasticised lumbar support or pregnancy shorts.
- Heat packs give relief to tight, aching muscles. Start gentle spinal stretches after the heat pack (you should feel muscle tightness but avoid deeper stretches for 12 to 16 weeks).
- Massage spinal and buttock muscles for relief of muscle tightness or spasms.
- Ensure baby's change table is high enough to prevent stooping.
- Place baby's bath on a bench to prevent bending over a low bathtub as lifting in the bent position risks straining spinal ligaments and muscles. Empty water before lifting the tub.
- Always bend the knees and hips to lift, while keeping the lower back straight and buttocks out behind (not curled under).
- When feeding baby in sitting, place one foot on a stool and hold baby close to avoid stooping.
- Use a lumbar cushion support in the chair when feeding baby or driving.
- *Avoid sit-ups or strenuous exercises and keep 'strengthening from the inside out'. Stay on track with the floor and core program and avoid exercises that isolate and strongly brace the upper abdomen.*
- Start regular walking and swimming (after bleeding stops) to engage spinal and core muscles. Begin with the *Shrink the Jellybelly* routine (page 155) to restore posture and progress PF and core muscular control.

Breastfeeding Positions

To avoid neck, shoulder and upper back pain while feeding, draw baby in close to the breast rather than bending down to feed. Choose an upright chair and avoid lounge chairs that place the spine in a 'C' curve position. Sitting up in bed for long feeding sessions causes slumping on the coccyx and sacrum, leading to discomfort and strain in the lower spine and sacroiliac joints.

- The side-lying position is ideal for breastfeeding directly after baby is born or following a caesarean birth.
- Sit tall; don't lean back away or slump forwards over baby. Support the lower back with a pillow.
- Breastfeeding is always an ideal time to work on a couple of sets of PF strength exercises while sitting tall. Repeat them in the standing position as well.
- The hormone controlling milk production is an appetite stimulant. Eating foods with a lower glycemic index (GI) helps to control hunger through slower release of energy and lower rises in insulin levels. See resources for GI information.
- Ask your midwife or lactation consultant to help with practising different positions and learning correct attachment so breast-feeding is a relaxing time.

Sharon Trotter, a leading U.K. midwife and mother and baby consultant gives the following advice–

'Regarding feeding positions, the important point to remember is that it is personal to each mother and she needs to experiment until she finds a position that works best for her and her baby. Keeping the baby's body in line with her own and close to her is vital as this increases skin-to-skin contact, thereby stimulating her to produce oxytocin, which in turn causes the nipples to become erect making it easier for the baby to attach to the breast.

Feeding is then more likely to be successful and the chance of sore nipples is reduced. There are a few standard positions like lying the baby across the abdomen, lying side by side in bed (ideal in the early days if the perineum is sore or after a c-section) or the rugby ball approach (holding the baby under your arm—good for premmies or to take the pressure off a sore nipple), but remember there are 360 degrees of attachment, so do what feels right for you and let your baby lead the way. Lying semi-prone is good, as well as letting your baby lie on your chest so they can self-attach using biological nurturing techniques.'

For further breastfeeding tips and techniques visit: tipslimited.com and biologicalnurturing.co.uk

Lifting

New mothers must avoid heavier activities or lifting older children as the weight is often too excessive for their PF muscle control. Swollen, stitched or bruised PF muscles will initially struggle to lift and support pelvic organs. If the deep core abdominal and spinal muscles are not engaging with the PF muscles during activity, the lower back and sacroiliac joints are at risk of being injured.

Avoid injury by:

- Beginning good postural habits in the early postpartum days by holding a tall posture with a small curve in the low back to keep PF and core muscles automatically active.
- Engaging PF muscles before lifting, use the 'knack' (page 21).
- Avoiding chest slumping and pushing your pelvis forwards when standing with baby.
- Asking for help with heavier tasks at home (lifting toddlers, heavy washing, bags of groceries, vacuuming, etc).
- Always lift with bent knees and hips while keeping the lower back flat and buttocks out behind, to engage long spinal strength

muscles.

- Avoiding working over low benches with a rounded spine as this position shuts down supporting core and trunk muscles.
- Stop any activity that causes the pelvic floor to descend.

Stomach Flattening Check

To flatten your stomach, stand tall; lift the PF muscles from underneath your body to engage the transversus abdominis, which acts like a corset to flatten the abdomen. Avoid sucking in the waist or clenching the buttocks.

Try this easy test to check if the PF muscles are leading the action.

Stand in front of a long bathroom mirror and lift up your PF muscles. A 'normal' abdominal reaction to a pelvic floor lift is slow tension back at the lower abdomen (transversus abdominis) with slight flattening of the abdomen. Waist tightening and narrowing, or buttock clenching, indicates that strong upper abdominal and buttock muscles are leading the action. Alternatively, lift the pelvic floor before making a long hissing sound, to observe the correct abdominal flattening action.

Women without incontinence automatically lift PF muscles first, with activity. One study showed women with stress incontinence switched on upper abdominal muscles first (external obliques) before their PF muscles (fig. 9). Even though their PF muscles were working hard, they were not able to prevent leaking with the rise of pressure inside the abdomen due to early upper abdominal muscle activity.

Tiredness

Fatigue is normal after vaginal birth and even greater following abdominal caesarean surgery. Having a baby is likely to be the biggest

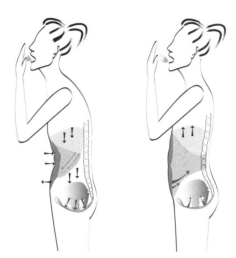

Fig. 9. Muscle activity of continent (right) and stress incontinent (left) women

life change you will ever experience and it may be difficult to adjust to the day-to-day stress of caring for a new baby. To counter the demands made on energy levels, take every opportunity to catch up on sleep.

Accept offers of help with cooking and housework to free up precious time to rest and bond with baby and partner. Reduce self-imposed stress by being realistic and forgiving as regards fitting into favourite jeans, keeping a spotless house or meeting other's expectations. Nurture yourself with fresh healthy food, baths, massages, favourite music and lots of cuddles.

Post Baby Blues and Depression

The blues can affect up to 80 per cent of new mothers in the first week after giving birth and usually disappears in a week or two. Getting more sleep and seeking help from family and friends are effective ways to overcome the blues.

Symptoms of postpartum depression in the first year after birth include feelings of anxiety, loss of interest in food, sex and other pleasurable activities, lasting longer than two weeks. Typical feelings are exhaustion, tearfulness and loss of confidence, inability to cope, memory problems, and sleep and appetite changes. These feelings are related to hormonal imbalance, sleep deprivation, exhaustion, body changes, postpartum pain and pelvic floor dysfunction.

Seek help and advice from health care providers early, as there are many proven ways to overcome depression. Sleep, exercise, counselling, problem solving therapy, interpersonal psychotherapy, cognitive behavior therapy, massage, meditation, diet, fish oils and some supplements are effective proven treatments. Women with moderate to severe PMS (pre menstrual syndrome), a history of depression or have suffered previous postpartum depression, are most at risk and require professional intervention.

When birth is traumatic or an unexpected caesarean is performed, a 'post traumatic' reaction may occur. Women who experience an unexpected or unwanted caesarean may grieve for the loss of a vaginal birth, leaving them feeling sad, anxious, violated or betrayed. The symptoms of any birth related trauma can emerge weeks, months or even years after the event. Talk to your midwife about how you are feeling before going home. Results from an Australian trial showed an early group exercise and education program for new mums lead by a physiotherapist, reduced the risk of postpartum depression among the intervention group.

If you or your partner become aware of any feelings associated with depression, speak with your caregivers early to ensure you receive guidance and if necessary, professional assistance. Counselling and support groups help to resolve frustration, anger, grief or resentment. Involve your partner so they can offer physical and emotional support and begin to understand what you are going through. When new mothers develop depression, their partners also have a higher risk of developing depressive symptoms. Visit The Black Dog Institute site below to take the 'Depression in pregnancy and postnatal self-test'.

For further information on postpartum depression visit:
panda.org.au,
beyondblue.org.au
blackdoginstitute.org.au

Early Postpartum

Key Points

- Fill out the New Mothers Pelvic Floor Questionnaire to record specific postpartum issues that are sometimes overlooked.
- Take the diastasis rectus test to check for abdominal muscle separation.
- Temporary loss of bladder control is common after vaginal and caesarean birth and responds well to committed PF exercises.
- The risk of prolapse is increased when pushing starts before the reflexive urge begins, the second stage of labour is prolonged, forceps or suction is required, or the first time mother is over 35.
- Use the 'knack' action to lift PF muscles before coughing or lifting.
- Always lift with bent hips and knees while keeping the lower back flat and buttocks out behind to engage long spinal strength muscles.
- Reduce self-imposed stress by being realistic and forgiving as regards fitting into favorite jeans, keeping a spotless house or meeting others expectations.
- Accept offers of help with cooking and housework to free up precious time to rest and bond with baby and partner.
- Post baby blues affect up to 80 per cent of new mothers in the first week after giving birth and usually disappear in a week or two.
- Sleep, exercise, counselling, problem solving therapy, interpersonal psychotherapy, cognitive behavior therapy, massage, meditation, diet, fish oils and some supplements are effective proven treatments for postnatal depression.

Early Postpartum questions to ask birth attendants:

SECTION 7

Recovery After Vaginal Birth

For the majority of pregnant women, a vaginal birth is the optimal and safest way to bring their baby into the world. It is a deeply enriching experience, bonding mother, baby and partner, when education, encouragement and guidance are provided. Support from positive partners and trusted caregivers in a comfortable, safe, calm environment makes an enormous difference in how a woman experiences vaginal birth. This section contains practical advice on recovering from specific pelvic floor or pelvic injuries following vaginal birth.

Skin, Perineal Muscle Tearing and Episiotomy

While it is common for first time mums to sustain a minor, first-degree tear, the perineal area has a rich blood supply and heals quickly. Third and fourth degree tears are rare and more likely (but not always) to be associated with an extension of an episiotomy. Trauma (grazes and tears) to the anterior genitals affects the labia, front vaginal wall, urethra or clitoris. Injury to the posterior perineum affects the back vaginal wall, perineal muscles, anal sphincters and lining of the bowel. Bruising may occur to the genitals during a forceps or ventous delivery.

There are different degrees of tearing:

- A first degree tear involves injury to the skin.
- A second degree tear extends into the perineal muscles.
- A third degree tear extends into part of or complete tearing of the anal sphincters.
- A fourth degree tear is a complete tear of the anal sphincters into the mucosa or lining of the bowel.

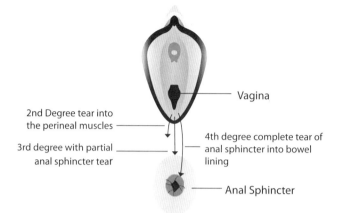

2nd Degree tear into
the perineal muscles

3rd degree with partial
anal sphincter tear

Vagina

4th degree complete tear of
anal sphincter into bowel
lining

Anal Sphincter

Fig 10. Perineal tears

Care for tears or stitches with the following actions:

- Each time you pass urine, fill a squirt (plastic sauce) bottle with warm water, squirt over the stitches and pat dry.
- Use ice packs over the stitched, swollen or bruised area for 10 to 15 minutes or massage with an ice block immediately after the birth for 5 to 10 minutes every 2 to 3 hours for 48 hours or until swelling reduces. *Try frozen pads to reduce perineal swelling.*
- Spend 15 to 30 minutes lying down each day without the pad to promote healing. Sunbaths of 10 to 15 minutes are recommended for healing if you are assured of privacy!
- Use a urinary alkaliniser e.g. Ural, to reduce stinging when passing urine. Cranberry juice reduces the incidence of urinary tract infections.
- Hold a clean pad or folded toilet paper against your perineum to protect stitches during bowel opening.
- Use a stool softener, eat foods with higher fibre content (especially soluble fibre found in fruit, legumes and vegetables)

and drink at least 6 glasses of water a day to keep stools soft.

- Some pain medication causes constipation. Rather than risk further muscle damage from straining, ask your midwife for stool softeners while taking pain medication.
- Change pads regularly and do not use tampons, which can introduce bacteria.
- Start gentle PF muscle exercises (quick tighten/relax) to improve pelvic circulation, reduce swelling and speed up healing. Do 10 repetitions, 5 times daily. Moving around improves general circulation.
- Watch for signs of infection around a tear or stitched area. Continued pain, tenderness, redness, abdominal pain, difficulty urinating, thick discharge, offensive smell and fever are signs of infection, which require antibiotics.

Adding support to the perineum with bowel opening (for 2 to 4 weeks) is important for all new mothers to reduce strain on recently stretched pelvic muscles and supports.

- Wear a firm pair of stretch briefs with a thick pad to keep pressure on the perineum.
- After the bowel empties, use wet wipes to clean the anal area from front to back.
- Avoid heavy lifting to minimise internal pressure increases down onto the pelvic floor.
- Use a soft cushion or pillow for comfortable sitting.
- Physiotherapists use ultrasound therapy over the perineum to reduce swelling and discomfort (24 to 36 hours postpartum).

Postpartum bleeding is typically constant for the first few days, before reducing to the regular menstrual loss. Initially, blood loss is bright red for 3 to 5 days and heavier than a normal period. It becomes pinker day 5 to 9 and creamy brown onwards. Light blood loss or spotting may continue for longer but this varies between women (may only be 2 to 3 weeks). Blood loss is initially augmented when breastfeeding helps to contract the uterus. Consult a midwife if you pass large clots or are concerned about blood loss.

Anal Sphincter Tears

Poor wind and stool control, bowel urgency and painful intercourse are signs of anal sphincter damage that may not be detected postpartum. Around 11 per cent of women experience faecal incontinence at 3 to 6 months after vaginal or caesarean birth.

When the internal anal sphincter is affected, leaking of bowel content is uncontrolled (passive incontinence). A tear into the external anal sphincter leaves a woman unable to clamp the sphincter shut and prevent loss of faecal matter (stress and urge incontinence).

If you experience any loss of wind or stool control, urgency or chronic constipation, request an endoanal ultrasound (to detect internal and external sphincter tears) and consult a gastro-enterologist.

Treatment involves early repair of sphincter rupture (with a surgeon skilled in sphincter repair), antibiotics, PF exercises, biofeedback and stool softeners or laxatives for easy bowel emptying. Sacral nerve stimulation is effective in the longer-term management of faecal incontinence. A small battery operated device is inserted over the sacrum to deliver impulses to the sacral nerves supplying the anal area.

Non-Surgical Early Treatment

- Reduce swelling by placing ice packs over the tear or repair for 10 to 15 minutes or use ice massage for 5 to 10 minutes, every 2 to 3 hours for 2 to 3 days.
- Take prescribed oral pain medication. Do not use pain

medication in a suppository form inserted in the bowel.

- Lie down for breastfeeding and avoid lifting more than baby for 4–6 weeks.
- Take fibre or prescribed softeners and extra water to soften the stools as pain medication has a constipating effect on bowel contents.
- If you are prone to constipation, continue using softening agents or bulking emulsions for 6 weeks or as long as required.
- Use a handheld shower spray to clean around the anus after bowel empting.
- Avoid sitting on a rubber ring as the circle of pressure restricts blood flow to and from the stitched area and slows healing.
- Start PF exercises when comfortable.
- Request ultrasound around the tear.
- Make an appointment to see a midwife or women's health physiotherapist before leaving hospital. They will provide dietary advice, sphincter exercises and biofeedback to ensure the success of a surgical repair.

Anal Fissures and Haemorrhoids

Early postpartum, anal fissures and/or haemorrhoids may present. These painful conditions are related to:

- Heavy birth weight babies.
- Traumatic labour or birth.
- Forceps to assist birth.
- Chronic constipation and difficulty with full bowel emptying.
- Tearing of the tissues around the anus.

Suggested actions:

- Soak in a warm bath several times a day (after stitches are removed). In hospital, small round tubs are placed in the toilet to take a mini bottom bath. Warm soaks relax the sphincters and increase blood flow to promote healing.

- Continue daily PF exercises and walk regularly.
- Avoid heavy lifting and prolonged coughing.
- Avoid straining or prolonged sitting to empty the bowel (use the position on page 34).
- Use wet wipes or a handheld shower spray to clean the anal area after the bowel empties. Toilet paper may be too abrasive to use.
- Treat constipation with a stool softener to avoid straining. Ask about a suitable non-chemical softener when taking medication or breastfeeding.
- Ask caregivers about prescribing corticosteroid foam, cream or suppository to relieve pain, inflammation, swelling and itching.
- *Combining medication with good anal hygiene and the listed suggestions will help shrink hemorrhoids and assist anal fissure healing.*

Coccyx Damage

Occasionally, childbirth (in a back lying or supported sitting position) causes damage to the coccyx where it attaches to the sacrum at the base of the spine. Some women report a 'popping' sound during birth and develop a painful coccyx postpartum.

The coccyx doesn't actually break; it consists of two or three segments linked by ligaments and childbirth or a fall onto the buttocks can weaken the connections between these segments. Sitting forces the weak joints apart, causing pain. Seek treatment if coccyx pain is aggravated by PF exercises, or if the joint does not heal and remains painful.

Coccyx injury, pain and discomfort may last from 6 to 12 months. Some women report relief after focal injections, while others resort to having the coccyx surgically removed (this does not always resolve the problem and post operative complications are common).

Suggested actions:

- Visit a doctor who specialises in coccyx injuries and a women's health physiotherapist to check the coccyx and sacral alignment. Muscle spasms and trigger points in PF muscles or buttock muscles attaching to the sacrum may be aggravating the coccyx pain and require myofascial release, stretching, dry needling or pain relieving injections.
- An x-ray or MRI scan will be suggested initially. Be sure to ask the radiographer for a clear view of the coccyx so it is included in the x-ray. Ask about a sit/stand dynamic x-ray to show if the coccyx is dislocating with sitting.
- Initially, use ice packs to reduce swelling along with anti-inflammatory and pain medication to relieve acute pain.
- Sit on a coccyx cushion to reduce pressure.
- Keep body weight over the sitting bones and the front pubic bone. It is usually more comfortable to sit in a slightly forward leaning position.

Continually leaning the weight to one side may aggravate bursitis around the hip taking all the weight.

- In the car, use the coccyx cushion underneath and a small support cushion in the lower back.
- Avoid sitting for long periods; stand and move frequently.
- Keep bowel movements soft to avoid straining.
- Pain may be prolonged if the muscles controlling the bladder are weak or not working effectively postpartum. After inflammation

reduces, learning to tighten and lift the PC muscle may ease pain for some sufferers in the short and long term. Begin this action gently to prevent aggravating pain.

- Some women gain relief of ongong pain after a focal ganglion impar block or injection into the sacrococcygeal junction by a doctor experienced in treating coccyx injuries.

Recovery After Vaginal Birth

Key Points

- While it is common for first time mums to sustain a minor, first-degree tear, the perineal area has a rich blood supply and heals quickly.
- Try frozen pads to reduce perineal swelling.
- Third and fourth degree tears are rare and more likely (but not always) to be associated with an extension of an episiotomy.
- Watch for signs of infection at the perineal tear or stitched area. Continued pain, tenderness, redness, abdominal pain, difficulty urinating, thick discharge, offensive smell and fever are signs of infection, which require antibiotics.
- Adding support to the perineum with bowel opening is important for all new mothers.
- The first two months postpartum are when anal fissures and/or haemorrhoids are more likely to develop.
- Poor wind and stool control, bowel urgency and painful intercourse are signs of anal sphincter damage that may not be detected postpartum.
- Combining medication with good anal hygiene and the listed suggestions will help shrink hemorrhoids and assist anal fissure healing.
- Occasionally, childbirth causes damage to the coccyx where it attaches to the sacrum at the base of the spine. Visit a doctor who specialises in coccyx injuries and a women's health physiotherapist to check the coccyx and sacral alignment.
- Some women gain relief of ongoing coccyx pain after a focal ganglion impar block or injection into the sacrococcygeal junction by a doctor experienced in treating coccyx injuries.

RecoveryAfter Vaginal Birth questions to ask birth attendants:

SECTION 8

Recovery After Caesarean Birth

Healing after surgery (along with enjoying and caring for your newborn) is now a priority. Accept offers of help with cooking, washing and housework from friends and family. Let them know beforehand how much you would value the gift of a few hours of their time with cooking, baby-sitting or housework.

Recovery rates vary between women following a caesarean, taking from three to six months for the uterus and deep abdominal muscle layers to fully heal, so allow time to regain abdominal strength and shape. Start with regular postural corrections, slow-paced walks and begin to slowly and gently strengthen from the inside out with the Shrink the Jellybelly routine when your scar feels more comfortable.

Immediately following a caesarean, time is spent in recovery while vital signs stabilise. It can take hours for the anesthetic to wear off and for feeling to return to the lower body. Ask for an extra heated blanket if shaking starts in the recovery period. Sometimes an annoying pain is felt under the shoulder blade caused by air entering the abdominal cavity during surgery. Wind pain is often experienced during the first few days (common after all abdominal surgery). Passing wind after surgery is a good sign showing the intestinal muscles are contracting to move gas along and out of the body. Headaches occasionally present after an epidural.

Compression stockings (TED stockings) are routinely worn postoperatively in hospital to lower the risk of deep vein thrombosis. While resting in bed, start simple leg exercises to improve circulation. Breathing exercises are important now to increase the exchange of oxygen and carbon dioxide.

Bed Exercises (lying on back)

- Pedal both feet up and down and circle ankles for 1 to 2 minutes.
- Gently lift PFMs as you breathe out; hold and release for five repetitions.
- Lift PFMs before sliding one heel up towards your buttock. Straighten and repeat for five repetitions with each leg. Be sure to breathe as you go.
- Bring both heels up toward your buttocks with feet resting on the bed. Gently flatten the lower back into the bed, then gently arch it upwards. Do five to ten easy repetitions.

Getting Out Of Bed

- Roll onto your side and lower both feet over the side of the bed with knees bent.
- Push into the bed using your uppermost hand at the same time as you lower your legs over the side of the bed—all in one smooth action.

To Protect Sutures When Coughing

- Place one hand on top of the other centrally over the scar and curl fingers around your pubic bone.
- Press both elbows firmly into your side.
- Lift your PFMs and cough.

The first 24 hours are challenging due to the restrictions of a urinary catheter (to drain the bladder) and an intravenous drip to administer fluid, pain medication and antibiotics if needed. The catheter and drip are usually removed the next day, which makes moving around somewhat easier. Bladder incisions (occur infrequently during caesareans) require an indwelling catheter for 7 to 10 days, which is associated with a higher rate of urinary tract infections. Inform carers if you have pain or problems urinating.

Some women report low levels of pain, while others need regular pain relief and more support following a surgical birth. Attitudes to pain, complications, the support received and coping skills with emotional issues determine the level of pain experienced post-surgery.

Drugs given during or after surgery for pain control can affect how the bladder (and bowel) works. Once the catheter is removed, empty the bladder every few hours for a day or two, as a full bladder may cause pressure and pain on the caesarean scar. Speak to carers if the regular sensations associated with a full bladder are not present.

To encourage urine flow, try a warm shower or pour water over the perineum to relax PF muscles. The first bowel movement can be a bit scary, with natural concern about putting pressure on the caesarean scar. Place the palm of your hand over the scar and apply gentle pressure while relaxing the abdomen and anal sphincter. Sitting tensed up on the toilet keeps the anal sphincter closed. As some pain relieving medication slows the bowel action, keep up water intake, eat fibre-rich foods and ask your midwife about stool softeners.

Vaginal blood losses are similar to losses after vaginal birth and are checked for the amount and colour of the blood. When baby is breastfed, their sucking releases hormones, initially causing uterine contractions to seal the uterus after placental detachment.

The length and amount of bleeding following caesarean or vaginal birth is related to the type of birth (less with physiological placental delivery), whether there was postpartum haemorrhage and the amount of rest a mother gets in the first month following birth. It's normal to pass some blood clots but check with your midwife after clots are passed.

Caring for the Caesarean Scar

It is wise to delay returning to activity and restrict the everyday workload for at least 6 weeks, to ensure healing is uninterrupted. Sutures hold the wound layers together while collagen repairs the abdominal and uterine incisions. The stitches dissolve later (or are removed) as tissue healing progresses.

Regularly check the scar for signs of infection: redness, pain, and local areas of tenderness, offensive smell, swelling or oozing of fluid. Even though antibiotics are routinely given in theatre, infection can still develop after surgery.

The scar is purple after surgery, taking months to go from purple to pink to white, and pubic hair re-growth may partly cover the scar. Gentle massage and scar stretching promotes healing and helps to prevent adhesions from forming between the uterus and other organs, but only once the scar is sufficiently healed. If massage is too firm or started too early, it will cause bleeding and slow healing.

Do not commence scar massage until you have clearance from your surgeon.

See page 139 for scar mobilising precautions and techniques. Avoid Brazilian waxing until perineal or abdominal scars are fully healed and pain free. Some women report numbness or hypersensitivity around the scar, which may take up to 12 to 24 months to regain normal sensation. Typical caesarean scar problems and suggested treatments are listed on page 138 (Table 1).

Suggested Actions:

- Within 24 hours you will be encouraged to get out of bed with assistance, if there are no complications. Pain medication is usually routinely prescribed, but always ask if more pain relief is needed so these early adventures are more tolerable. A shower relaxes and freshens and walking upright helps to pass abdominal wind, improves circulation and reduces the risk of deep vein thrombosis.

- Support the scar with your palm while getting out of bed and walking to the bathroom. Roll onto your side and use the other arm to push up. Hold your abdomen when coughing or sneezing.

- *Instead of coughing, use repeated 'huffing' to dislodge any chest secretions and reduce the impact of strong coughing on the scar. This is like fogging up a mirror as you huff out. Repeat 3 to 4 times then cough (with support) if there is something loose to expel.*

- It is safe to shower with a waterproof dressing and once the dressing is removed, gently run water over the incision line, but avoid using soap. Pat dry with a fresh towel. Sometimes silicone tape is placed over the incision line and changed daily for 2 to 4 weeks to decrease scarring. Hydrocolloidal dressings (Duoderm) are also used to improve scar healing.

- Wear high-waisted knickers (Bridget Jones style) to avoid the elastic top rubbing on or irritating the incision line.

- Place a pad over the scar (stick to the knickers) to prevent them rubbing on the stitches.

- Pay attention to 'tall' sitting, standing and walking postures. Breathe out as you sit or stand up into a 'tall' posture.

- Start gentle PF exercises to engage the deep abdominal muscle and lift PF muscles before picking up baby.

Vaginal Birth After Caesarean Section

Vaginal birth after caesarean (VBAC) is an attractive option to many women who previously birthed by caesarean, as success rates for VBAC are now 60 per cent to 80 per cent with a supported team approach. Discussion of the individual risks associated with a VBAC or subsequent caesarean will help with the decision to undergo a trial of labour.

Each additional caesarean increases future placental problems as well as the risk of uterine rupture—a risk of less than one per cent with a lower uterine incision and around 10 per cent with a vertical, upper uterine incision. Following caesarean birth, there is a slightly higher risk of uterine rupture during subsequent pregnancies, both with a VBAC or a repeat elective caesarean birth.

The obstetric history and maternal characteristics are used to determine a woman's chances of success with a VBAC. Predictors of VBAC success are: previous vaginal delivery, previous VBAC, spontaneous labour, the degree of cervical dilation on initial labour presentation, inter pregnancy interval of more than 18 months and a pre-term birth.

The chances of a successful VBAC are decreased with the following presentations: maternal obesity, short stature, the maternal age is over 40, the gestational age is over 41 weeks, increased weight gain between pregnancies, diabetes before or during pregnancy and disproportional foetal head to pelvis size.

The risk of uterine rupture during VBAC is decreased with: spontaneous labour, a previous vaginal birth, pre-term labour and the interval between pregnancies is over 18 months. The risk of uterine rupture is increased with: a prior vertical incision caesarean, two or more caesareans, single layer closure of the uterus, induction of labour, use of prostaglandins, infection of previous caesarean wound and a shorter interval between pregnancies.

Short term caesarean risks and complications associated with anesthesia include: blood clots, pulmonary embolism and wound infection. Longer term risks include miscarriage, a low-lying placenta (previa) or placenta growing into the uterus (accreta) and premature birth. The risk of placenta previa and accreta directly increases with the number of previous caesarean sections. Reduced fertility related to post caesarean adhesions affects approximately 10 per cent of women.

A previous caesarean with or without labour does not affect the uterus's ability to labour, and a VBAC labour advances the same as a regular vaginal birth. If labour stops or slows down and there is no physical cause, the reason could be anxiety or fear. Being surrounded by trusted people offering support and guidance helps the mother work through this stage. For further information on VBAC visit:

canaustralia.net
cares-sa.org.au
birthrites.org

Recovery After Caesarean Birth

Key Points

- Immediately following a caesarean, time is spent in recovery while vital signs stabilise. It can take hours for the anaesthetic to wear off and for feeling to return to the lower body.
- The first 24 hours are challenging due to the restrictions of a urinary catheter (to drain the bladder) and an intravenous drip to administer fluid, pain medication and antibiotics if needed.
- It is wise to delay returning to activity and restrict the everyday workload for at least 6 weeks, to ensure healing of the scar is uninterrupted.
- Do not commence scar massage until you have clearance from your surgeon.
- Avoid Brazilian waxing until abdominal scars are fully healed and pain free.
- Support the scar with your palm while getting out of bed and walking to the bathroom. Roll onto your side and use the other arm to push up.
- Vaginal birth after caesarean (VBAC) should be considered when a woman has previously birthed by caesarean.
- The obstetric history and maternal characteristics are used to determine a woman's chances of success with a VBAC.
- A previous caesarean with or without labour does not affect the uterus's ability to labour, and a VBAC labour advances the same as vaginal birth.
- Reduced fertility related to post caesarean adhesions affects approximately 10 per cent of women.

Recovery after Caesarean Birth questions to ask birth attendants:

SECTION 9

Pelvic Floor Self Assessment

Pelvic floor external and internal self-examination 5–6 weeks after baby is born uncovers tender, tight or hypersensitive areas along with signs of prolapse. Before resuming intercourse, relieve concerns about how intimacy will feel, by taking your own vaginal tour.

The vagina is a long fibromuscular tube situated behind the bladder and in front of the rectum, and extends from the uterus to the vulva. When a woman stands, the vagina points in an upward and backward direction and the sides are normally in contact. It has an internal mucosal lining and a muscular layer with an outer layer of circular muscles and an inner layer of longitudinal muscles.

The rich vaginal blood supply promotes good repair of muscle lacerations and tears. The lower third of the vagina has a higher number of nerve endings, making it more sensitive than the upper two thirds. If you don't wish to self-examine, consult a women's health physiotherapist, medical specialist or general practitioner.

Pelvic floor self-assessment consists of four examination elements each of which is discussed in the following pages.

1. **External genital skin changes or scars**

2. **Vaginal pain and scars**

3. **PF muscle/tendon damage at pubic symphysis**

4. **Vaginal pelvic organ prolapse**

External Genital Skin Changes or Scars

Initially, position a mirror under the pelvic floor and with clean hands, feel the skin over your clitoris, outer and inner labia, and vaginal opening. Look for scars, lesions and irritated red skin. Feel the perineum (the area between the anus and vagina) to see if it moves side to side, and up and down, the same on each side. Make a note of any changes in skin colour, sensitivity, lesions or an area of restricted skin movement.

Vaginal Pain and Scars

Begin the vaginal exploration with one or two fingers inserted up to the first finger joint (Fig.11). Use lubrication if needed.

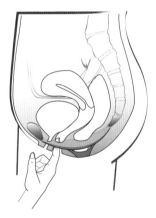
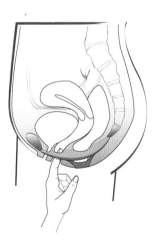

Fig. 11. Lower 1/3 vaginal palpation
(front and back walls)

Think of an imaginary clock face on your pelvic floor with the clitoris at 12 o'clock and the back of the vagina at 6 o'clock. Begin at the pubic bone and slowly sweep your finger/s around one way in a half circle, then back to the starting point to complete the other half circle. Feel for tender areas, tight muscles and bands of scar tissue. The lower third of the vagina is enclosed by the levator ani muscles and the bulbocavernosus muscle surrounds the vaginal opening.

The front vaginal wall feels 'rough' or slightly ridgy. Around 4–6 centimeters into the vaginal entrance is a slightly sensitive area: this is the G spot where the urethra and vagina form a vaginal erogenous zone. The spot is easier to find when fully aroused and stimulation without arousal may cause discomfort.

Move your fingers deeper (past the second joints on your fingers) and repeat the same circles. The upper vagina is more capacious, stretchy and less sensitive than the lower area. You may need to reach a little higher to feel your firmer cervix sitting at the top of the vagina.

After completing each of the lower and upper sweeps, write down the location and pain intensity of any painful, tight or hypersensitive areas e.g. Outer sweep—tender ridge at 5.00 o'clock, left side, 7/10 pain. Inner sweep; tender 7.00 o'clock right side, 4/10 pain. Keep light pressure over any tender area for 30–60 seconds to guage if the tenderness subsides.

Pelvic Floor Tendon/Muscle Damage

Magnetic Resonance Imaging and Transperineal Ultrasound are used to detect if the levator ani muscles have separated from their attachment to the pubic bone. Researchers have identified a higher risk of muscle damage with assisted births using rotational forceps, particularly in first time mothers over 35 years. If the tendon (which joins muscle to bone) separates from one or both sides of the pubic bone, the muscles will be weaker or unable to contract. This injury is associated with anterior vaginal wall prolapse, which has a higher re-prolapse rate after surgical repair (in women with torn levator ani tendon attachments).

Not all women with PF muscle tendon separation experience urine loss or symptomatic prolapse. Two effective ways to self-detect tendon separation from the pubic bones are described below.

- Use a mirror to see what happens to your anal sphincter when it tightens, lifts and becomes smaller. If the sphincter skews to one side on the lift, this indicates levator ani tendon separation from the pubic bone on the opposite side.
- Insert both index or middle fingers vaginally and place them either side of the pubic bones (at 11 and 1 on a clock face).

Lift the PF muscles to feel the tendons firm under your fingers. If no firming is felt under one or both fingers, suspect a separation.

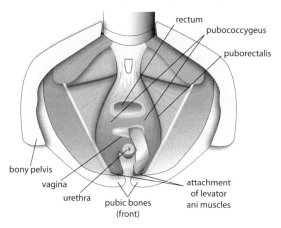

rectum
pubococcygeus
puborectalis
bony pelvis
vagina
urethra
pubic bones
(front)
attachment
of levator
ani muscles

Fig. 12. Palpating for musculotendinous
separation at pubic bone

Throughout the body, muscles are attached to bones via their tendons. Sometimes, strong force causes separation from the bone and/or damage at the junction between muscle and tendon or within the muscle belly. This damage is often partial and responds to muscle retraining. Although trials are underway, complete PF tendon rupture currently has no long-term successful surgical repair. Consult a gyneacologist or women's health physiotherapist for confirmation of findings; modify activity, develop protective pelvic habits and strengthen PF and core exercises to prevent future problems.

Identifying Vaginal Pelvic Organ Prolapse

Start by reviewing the different types of vaginal prolapse on page 94. Self-examination for prolapse is done in supported lying and standing, with one foot on a stool so gravity helps with assessment. Keep a pad and pen close to note any findings.

- Empty your bladder first and be conscious of relaxing PF muscles during the examination.
- Cough strongly and using a mirror, look for movement of a vaginal wall down to or out of the vaginal entrance. Note if a smooth bulge balloons more to the front or back of your vagina or if the firmer cervix is descending.
- Bear down firmly (pelvic floor relaxed) for 6 seconds, looking for any movement down to or out of the vaginal walls.
- If the cervix or a vaginal wall protrudes like a golf or tennis ball shape, this is a significant prolapse. When the prolapse skews more to one side, a levator ani tendon tear (from the pubic bone) is suspected. When a vaginal wall bulges into your inserted fingers (and not out of the vaginal entrance), the prolapse is contained internally.

Cervix/uterine descent:

Insert 1 or 2 fingers and note how many finger joints penetrate before feeling the firm cervix at the top of the vagina (feels like a dimpled chin). If the cervix is descended, push it upwards to gauge how far it lifts. Note how far it descends with coughing, then bearing down.

Next time, tighten and lift PF muscles first to determine if this action lifts or pushes the cervix down. If the cervix descends, a bearing down action is being used, instead of a lifting action. If the PF muscles feel strong and coordinated during the lift, the utero vaginal prolapse is more likely due to damage of supporting ligaments and connective tissue (rather than muscle weakness).

Anterior (front) vaginal wall prolapse:

Insert 1 or 2 fingers and place over the front vaginal wall (facing the bladder) to feel any bulging under your fingers, first with strong coughing and then with bearing down. A definite bulge of the wall under your fingers indicates a front vaginal wall prolapse.

Next, tighten the PF muscles before coughing to gauge if this action controls the front wall bulging.

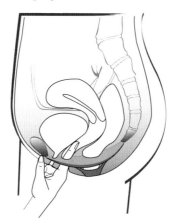

Fig. 13. Feeling for front wall prolapse

Posterior (back) vaginal wall prolapse:

Insert 1 or 2 fingers and place over the back vaginal wall (facing the rectum), to feel any bulging under your fingers, first with strong coughing and then with bearing down. A definite bulge under your fingers indicates a back vaginal wall prolapse.

Next, tighten the PF muscles before coughing to gauge if this action controls the back wall bulging.

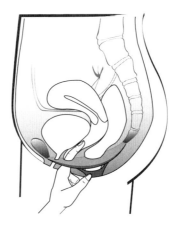

Fig. 14. Feeling for back wall prolapse

To identify a small intestinal prolapse, hold a tongue depressor (looks like a thick ice cream stick) over the back vaginal wall and reach your fingers up to the top of the back wall. Repeat the coughing and bearing down tests. The small intestinal prolapse presents with the upper back vaginal wall (the area between the back wall and cervix) descending down from above the depressor.

Discuss any positive findings with a gynaecologist and women's health physiotherapist to determine suitable treatment options.

Pelvic Floor Self Assessment

Key Points

- Before resuming intercourse, relieve concerns about how intimacy will feel by taking your own vaginal tour.
- Pelvic floor external and internal self-examination 5–6 weeks after baby is born uncovers tender, tight or hypersensitive areas along with any signs of prolapse.
- The rich vaginal blood supply promotes good repair of muscle lacerations and tears.
- The lower third of the vagina has a higher number of nerve endings, making it more sensitive than the upper two thirds.
- Pelvic floor self-assessment consists of 4 different sections to examine for: external genital skin changes; vaginal pain and scars; muscle/tendon damage at the pubic symphysis and identifying vaginal pelvic organ prolapse.
- Magnetic Resonance Imaging, Transperineal Ultrasound and palpation are used to detect if the levator ani muscles have separated from their attachment to the pubic bone.
- When the cervix or a vaginal wall protrudes like a golf or tennis ball shape with coughing, a significant prolapse is present.
- When the prolapse skews more to one side with coughing, a levator ani tendon detachment (from the pubic bone) is suspected.
- When a vaginal wall bulges into your inserted fingers (and not out of the vaginal entrance), the prolapse is contained internally.
- If any problems have been found, they can be treated. Seek help.

Pelvic Floor Self Assessment questions to ask caregivers:

SECTION 10

Caesarean Scars, Episiotomies and Perineal Tears

Following episiotomy, vaginal or perineal tears, most women heal uneventfully, however studies show the majority of women develop adhesions after pelvic surgery. Adhesions are bands of collagen the body produces to start healing immediately after surgery, infection, inflammation or trauma. Scar tissue forms in the external scar and adhesions form internally.

Complications occur when adhesions cause tension and restricted mobility between internal structures that are not usually connected. Post-surgical adhesions joining any area in the pelvis or abdomen to another structure (muscles, organs, bones, nerves, blood vessels) are likely to cause unusual pain and dysfunction.

In future pregnancies, pain may be felt as the growing uterus stretches and breaks adhesions between the uterus, other organs or the abdominal wall. The risk of placental attachment to the uterine scar site increases with each caesarean birth; making the surgery more complicated with increased time spent dividing scarring and adhesions from prior surgery.

Adhesions between the uterus, ovaries or fallopian tubes cause pelvic, back and intercourse pain and infertility when the egg and sperm are obstructed from travelling along the tube. Adhesions forming around the small intestine cause pain, diarrhoea, constipation or an irritable bowel and occasionally, obstruction.

Scar Issues in table 1 outlines treatment options for problematic caesarean scars. A multi disciplinary approach is most effective to heal problematic scars and prevent further complications from developing.

Scar issue	Symptoms	Treatment
Pain, infection.	Redness, oozing, swelling, bad odour, fever.	Immediately see caregiver – take antibiotics.
Pelvic, abdominal wall or uterine adhesions.	Pulling pain worse on quick standing or exercise. Difficult to stand tall. Painful intercourse.	Scar mobilisation techniques. Laparoscopy to remove adhesions. Ultrasound, laser.
Pain, scar endometriosis.	Ongoing monthly pain, shooting pain, bent posture.	Pain relief patches, medication and excision.
Scar hyper-sensitivity.	Scar sensitivity to touch or temperature.	Massage, injections and pain patches.
Scar patches of numbness.	Numb areas of skin around the scar.	Scar mobilisation techniques, allow time for nerve regrowth.
Raised keloid, discoloured scar.	Purple, raised areas.	Medical grade silicone sheets for 8–12 weeks. Duoderm patches.
Scar trigger points.	Deep local and referred pain on pressure.	Sustained pressure over trigger point, dry needling, injection, stretching.
Scar hernia.	Bulge or protrusion along the scar line.	Avoid lifting, wear compression garment, surgery.
Scar overhang.	Tight scar with abdominal fat overhang.	Early scar mobilisation, weight loss, scar revision or tummy tuck surgery.

Table 1. Caesarean Scar Problems and Management

Different soft tissue techniques are used to mobilise scars and prevent deeper adhesive bands from attaching to internal structures and pelvic organs. Some of the many techniques used are included in the following pages.

After gaining clearance from your surgeon, start slowly and gently mobilizing the scar to prevent tough scars and adhesions and improve blood circulation.

I encourage you to visit your caregiver and a therapist skilled in myofascial release for assessment and ongoing treatment with longer term or complicated scar issues.

Guidelines For Caesarean Scar Mobilisation.

CLEAR WITH SURGEON

Always ask your surgeon for approval and written guidelines before starting the mobilizing techniques.

PRECAUTIONS

Do not commence the techniques if scars or tears are oozing, bleeding, infected or have recently increased pain levels. Wait until vaginal bleeding ceases before mobilising perineal scars.

SEEK TREATMENT

Seek treatment immediately for any signs of scar discharge or infection.

BE GENTLE

Start techniques gently with light pressure and gradually increase stretching pressure over the following two to four weeks.

HOW TO BEGIN

Lie on your bed with head and shoulders supported and knees bent up.

FEEL THE SCAR

Start by slowly running fingers above and below the length of the scar, looking for areas of pain, numbness or hypersensitivity. Stay on a painful spot for 30–60 seconds until the pain eases. The local pain should ease when the pressure is repeated.

Caesarean Scar Mobilising Skills

Finger Strokes

Start by placing your index finger above and middle finger below the scar; slowly slide the fingers one way, and then reverse the direction back along the scar. Repeat 2 or 3 times.

Begin with light pressure and gradually increase pressure (never aggressive) for 60 seconds. Keep abdominal muscles relaxed.

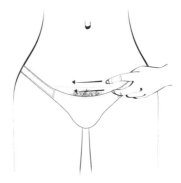

Fig. 13. Stroking

Small Figure 8s

Keep index and middle fingers together and start at one end by drawing small figures of 8's along the length of the scar then back in the reverse direction for 60 seconds. Repeat 2 or 3 times.

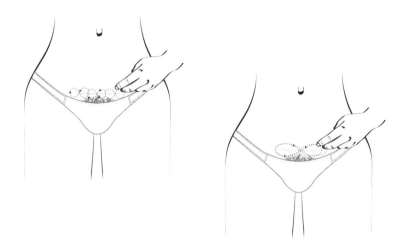

Continue these two techniques for 1–2 weeks (after gaining surgeon's approval) before adding more advanced scar mobilisation.

Advanced Scar Mobilisation

Scar Kneading

Spread all fingertips out underneath the scar and gently lift in the direction of the navel. Place both thumbs above the scar and slowly stretch down in the direction of the pubic bone using a kneading action. Repeat slowly for 60 seconds for 2 or 3 repetitions.

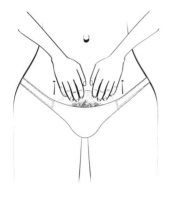
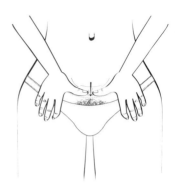

Fig. 15. Kneading

Scar Lifting

Place the index and middle fingers under and thumb above the scar. Gently pinch and lift the scar away from the body until you feel a stretch. Hold for 20–30 seconds. Repeat along the length of the scar for 2 or 3 repetitions.

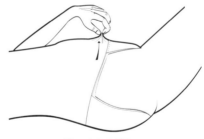

Fig. 16. Lifting

S–Stretches

Start at one end with the thumb of one hand above and index and middle fingers of the other hand below the scar. Lift the scar with the underneath finger tips *as* you push down with the thumb to form an S shape in the scar. Repeat in both directions for 60 seconds for 2 or 3 repetitions.

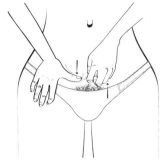

Fig. 17. S–Stretches

Hypersensitive Scars

Scar hypersensitivity and burning is related to new nerve endings that grow after surgery and over react to a sensation or temperature change that would not normally cause pain. Rather than avoiding any touch over the scar, add more stimuli to de-sensitise the new nerve endings.

Ultrasound therapy can help, as can topical agents such as capsaicin cream throughout the day or ask your caregiver to prescribe pain relief patches. Scar desensitizing injections of local anaesthetic and steroids help to reduce symptoms. Some women gain relief by regularly using a TENS machine.

Light finger moves

Place the index finger above and middle finger below one end of the scar and lightly tip tap along the scar in both directions for 20 to 30 seconds and repeat 2–3 times. Gradually increase pressure to build more tolerance to touch.

Finger circles

Place the index and middle fingers at one end of the scar and lightly circle along the scar in both directions. Repeat for 20 to 30 seconds, 2 to 3 times and gradually increase the pressure.

Brushing

Using a soft brush then a washcloth to stroke along the length of the scar with increasing pressure for 20/30/60 seconds. As hypersensitivity reduces, stroke with a firmer brush.

Perineal Scars

Use a mirror to check the perineal skin is healed and do not commence the techniques if any signs of infection, oozing, swelling or bleeding are present. Use Vitamin E, rose oil or other cold pressed oils to massage around the vulva and perineum. Avoid using scented soaps, feminine sprays or scented, coloured toilet paper. Gently stretch the scar up and down and side to side. Use the same pregnancy perineal massage technique (page 49) to mobilise scars after vaginal bleeding has stopped. Seek clearance before commencing perineal scar mobilisation (usually after 8 to 10 weeks) and begin with gentle stretching pressure.

If tender or tight areas were uncovered during your vaginal tour, slowly increase fingertip pressure over the area for 60 seconds before repeating a second time. Tight bands respond to very slow stretching pressure, cross wise along the length of the band for 20 to 30 second intervals until the band begins to soften (like a slow strumming with index and middle fingers). If the vagina is dry or an area is too sensitive to touch, an oestrogen tablet or cream may be prescribed.

Occasionally, the cumulative effect of nerve and muscle damage, stitches or perineal trauma, plus emotional trauma or fear, overloads the nervous system and triggers off a vulval pain syndrome (the term for different painful conditions in the vulval–vaginal area). Seek early treatment if conditions present.

Caesarean Scars, Episiotomies and Perineal Tears

Key Points

- Following episiotomy, vaginal or perineal tears, most women heal uneventfully, however studies show the majority of women develop adhesions after pelvic surgery.

- Complications occur when adhesions cause tension and restricted mobility between internal structures that are not usually connected.

- The risk of placental attachment to the uterine scar site increases with each caesarean, making the surgery more complicated for the surgeon with increased time spent dividing scarring and adhesions from prior surgery.

- Different soft tissue techniques are used to gently mobilise scars and prevent deeper adhesive bands from attaching to internal structures and pelvic organs.

- Always ask your surgeon for approval and written guidelines before starting the mobilising techniques.

- Do not commence scar techniques if scars or tears are oozing, bleeding, infected or pain has recently increased.

- Wait until vaginal bleeding ceases before mobilising perineal tears.

- Occasionally, the accumulative effect of nerve and muscle damage, stitches or perineal trauma, plus emotional trauma or fear, overloads the nervous system and triggers off a vulval pain syndrome (the term for different painful conditions in the vulval–vaginal area). Seek early treatment if conditions present.

Scar Questions to ask caregivers:

SECTION 11

Sex after Childbirth

Some women enjoy sex even more after their baby is born, while others feel anxious about or disinterested in sex for a variety of reasons. Libido levels are affected by lack of sleep, pain, and hormonal changes with breastfeeding, depressed mood and body changes. Breastfeeding stimulates prolactin (to increase milk production) but inhibits the release of oestrogen and progesterone needed for vaginal lubrication and libido.

Following a vaginal birth, skin abrasions and muscle tears are usually well healed by the six-week check-up, as the vagina and vulva have a rich blood supply. This usually means sex can recommence, but only if you are comfortable and pain-free. Wait until blood loss has ceased before resuming sex to ensure the placental wound inside the uterus has fully healed, thereby minimising the chance of infection entering the uterus.

Give your body time to heal after a caesarean or vaginal birth before resuming sex. Pain with postpartum sexual penetration is associated with caesarean section, episiotomy, perineal and anal sphincter tearing, coccyx damage, and stretching of pelvic nerves if the second stage was prolonged. **Pain and pressure on any wound leads to anxiety; so discuss feelings or fears with your partner who needs to be prepared to stop if you are uncomfortable.**

Studies show women's sexual health issues are common 6 months postpartum, regardless of the mode of birth. Six months following birth, one in five mother's reported pain with intercourse, and up to one in nine had not resumed sexual activity. Women who sustained anal sphincter tears were less likely to report sexual activity. Few women in the studies reported the pain or sought treatment for their symptoms. It is not normal to experience ongoing sexual pain months after childbirth; putting up with pain ruins sexual pleasure, bringing on apprehension and fear of intercourse for both partners.

In *Where Did My Libido Go*, Dr Rosie King guides women (and their partners) with low or lost libido on how to maximise their desire and arousal along with advice on getting their sex life back on track.

Reconnecting Sexually with Your Partner

Following surgery, tearing, stitches or pelvic pain, sexual self-confidence can take a dive. Some women take 6 to 12 months before feeling comfortable and confident to resume penetrative sexual activity. The following suggestions may help:

- Ask for partner pampering with foot rubs and back massages without the expectation of sex.
- Enjoy the relaxation of a bath with scented candles.
- Buy lingerie to reward your post baby body.
- Remember to frequently hug and kiss your partner, as it's easy to fill up cuddle quotas with baby.
- Go on date nights.
- Gently massage healed scars with Vitamin E, rose or almond oils to reconnect with your abdomen and perineum.
- Massage your uterus (located above the pubic bone and bladder), while sending positive loving thoughts and feeling pride in your abdomen and pelvis. The uterus usually regains its normal size 6 to 8 weeks after baby is born.
- Gentle abdominal massage by a therapist or your partner, improves blood flow to tummy muscles as they shorten and strengthen with exercise and activity.
- Engage in non-penetrative sexual activity to allow time for

healing of sensitive tissues.

- Only resume intercourse when your perineum, lower abdomen and vagina are pain free. Take your own vaginal tour as described on page 129 to discover the location of any sensitive areas prior to resuming penetrative sex.
- If breastfeeding reduces vaginal secretions, relieve discomfort during intercourse by using water-based lubricants or a cold pressed oil. Use a paraben free, non-petroleum based lubricant.
- Try new positions to prevent pressure on a caesarean scar and let your partner know if you don't want to be touched over the lower abdomen due to tenderness or sensitivity.
- Repeat regular PF exercises to recover muscle strength and orgasmic sensation. Urine loss with intercourse or less orgasmic sensation indicates that PF muscles lack coordination and strength.
- Stretch marks gradually narrow with time to finer, white lines. If they are still prominent six months postpartum, speak to a cosmetic doctor about using a vitamin A cream or dermabrasion.
- If practicing anal sex following an anal sphincter tear or repair, be guided by the surgeon as regards healing times. Risks associated with anal intercourse are disruption of sensitive rectal mucosa, bursting of haemorrhoids and anal cancer (linked to infection by the human papilloma virus).

Consult a gynaecologist and women's health physiotherapist for advice and treatment of sexual, pelvic or pelvic floor pain. For further information on pelvic pain visit:

pelvicpain.org
vaginismus.com

Vaginal Exercisers

Clients often enquire about using one of the wide varieties of pelvic floor exercisers, biofeedback machines, muscle stimulators or toners available to help complement PF muscle training. Vaginal exercisers provide feedback and resistance and if used regularly, can be effective to improve strength. Some manufacturers make great claims about their benefits and it is wise to ask for studies and research regarding the effectiveness of any device. The device must be made from medical grade plastic or silicone to be safe for vaginal use. If you are experiencing PF weakness, ask a women's health physiotherapist if a device is suitable for home use.

Biofeedback machines use a vaginally inserted probe connected to a monitor displaying the strength of the PF muscle contraction. The biofeedback gives visual or auditory feedback and encourages a higher level of muscular contraction. Learn the correct action before using a biofeedback to avoid becoming proficient with an incorrect action. Some biofeedbacks come with adjustable resistance and vaginal sensors in different sizes. A physiotherapist will explain the fitting and use of a biofeedback for home use and monitor progress between appointments. Biofeedback is also used to facilitate muscle relaxation in women with overactive PF muscles.

Pelvic floor muscle stimulators emit mild electrical currents via a vaginal probe or external electrodes, to stimulate muscle and nerve fibres in poorly functioning PF muscles. They are used to treat bladder urgency, stress and urge incontinence, frequency, bowel incontinence, and to improve PF muscle strength and endurance. While stimulators may be a valuable part of early treatment, they are not a long-term replacement for voluntary muscular control.

Vaginal weights are cones or balls of various weights inserted and retained vaginally. Keeping the weight from falling out requires PF muscle contraction while you stand and walk. Lighter–weight cones are used initially and replaced with slightly heavier cones as the PF muscles strengthen. The weights are best used in conjunction with PF exercises and are not effective in some women with prolapse. The cone can lodge in a vaginal position with no muscle lift required to stay in place, or it slips out immediately due to vaginal wall prolapse.

Incontinence devices are inserted vaginally under the bladder neck to control stress incontinence with exercise, allowing leak free activity. Gentle pressure by the device on the urethra controls urine loss. Use in conjunction with a PF exercise program to regain muscular function. A newer medical grade silicone device called *Incostress* (looks like a silicone tampon) is reusable for six months. It is also effective for strengthening when PF muscles are contracted to retain the incostress vaginally, while trying to draw it out. Read more at incostress.com

Pelvic toners are devices with two hinges that are held together when inserted (or removed) vaginally and open when hand pressure is removed. Tightening PF muscles squeezes the sides together. The toner must have a 'stop' feature to prevent it from fully closing and pinching the vulva or vagina. This device is unsuitable for women with tight PF muscles.

Dilators are used to stretch vaginal muscles to allow for more comfortable intercourse when tight PF muscles cause pain and prevent sexual penetration. Starting with a smaller sized dilator and using warmth for muscle relaxation, consistent use stretches the vaginal muscles before progressing to the next sized dilator. When trigger points are present in PF muscles, a dilator can be used to apply pressure over the internal trigger point to relieve pain.

SECTION 12

Return to Postpartum Exercise

Don't despair if your tummy is soft and floppy after baby is born, as all the abdominal muscles stretched to their outer range during pregnancy. Your body has undergone a sudden major change from having muscles tightly stretched over an expanded uterus, to a softer abdomen with weaker muscular control. Stretching and separation of the rectus abdominis muscles might leave you wondering what on earth has happened to your abdominal muscles, but they do shrink back with commitment to suitable exercises.

The smaller PF muscles in the base of the abdominal cylinder provided uplifting support during pregnancy and were stretched to extreme limits during birth. Reclaim a strong body by strengthening the pelvic floor first, in combination with the abdominals to fast track pelvic and trunk control. As PF and core muscles work most efficiently in their inner or 'shortened' position, exercising from the inside tightens and firms inner and outer abdominal muscles together.

Challenging abdominal exercises in the first 6 months postpartum are likely to overwhelm the control of smaller PF muscles. Avoid exercises that isolate abdominal muscles as these exercises do little to develop core function and dynamic stability. Practising PF and core exercises reduces abdominal muscle separation, whereas repeating sit-ups and sustained trunk curling pulls the abdominal separation apart.

Following a caesarean or complicated vaginal birth, start the early PF and core exercises when you are comfortable. Wear a support garment for the first 4–6 weeks (longer if needed) to support the pelvis and lower back, compress organs and improve posture.

Always report any pain experienced during exercise and seek guidance to check if you are doing the exercises correctly. Repeat the exercises slowly with an emphasis on using and controlling the PF and core muscles. Avoid rushing or doing them with force.

Exercise Guidelines

Focus on walking and holding upright postures in the first weeks after birth as you rebuild and retrain from 'the inside out' with pelvic floor and core exercises. Training inner muscles **first**—to recover strength and coordination—is the number one priority *before* starting aerobic, fitness or gym programs. Once you have an established routine of PF exercises, incorporate them into your own exercise programs to ensure pelvic floor protection throughout your life.

Time frames for resuming exercise are individual and depend on the level of fitness, exercise history, prior injuries or complications with birth and whether PF, core and trunk muscle rehabilitation has been consistent and effective. Be wary of returning straight to challenging exercise classes. For example, 'Bootcamp' is based on the Royal Canadian Air Forces 5BX and 10BX systems used for military personnel training and are not suitable for new mothers.

The following return to exercise guidelines contains suggested time frames for resuming aerobic activity, following an uncomplicated vaginal birth. Canadian clinical guidelines advise that moderate exercise during lactation does not affect the quantity or composition of breast milk or impact on infant growth.

Birth to 16 weeks—tall sitting, standing and walking, Shrink the Jellybelly exercises (page 155), Train It exercises (page 163), and easy swimming after blood loss has ceased.

16 to 24 weeks—postpartum exercise classes, low impact aerobic activities e.g. swimming, water aerobics, tai chi, basic belly dancing and Train It exercises.

24 weeks onwards—modified yoga, basic pilates and fit ball classes with experienced postpartum instructors.

Following a caesarean or complicated vaginal birth, commence the Shrink the Jellybelly program when you are comfortable, and gradually add easy activities as pain settles and your pelvis and trunk strengthens. Delay returning to more challenging physical activity for 6 to 12 months following a caesarean birth, third and fourth degree perineal tears, infection and further surgery, prolonged second stage with interventions, diastasis rectus separation, unresolved PGP, coccyx damage, prolapse and incontinence. Consult a women's health professional to guide activity according to your level of PF and core strength and general fitness.

Running

Avoid high-impact activities in the first 4 to 5 months until joints are more stable and PF and core muscles are stronger. Running is not suitable as an early activity due to the stress on joints and pelvic floor and the potential to cause discomfort in lactating breasts. Expressing or breast-feeding before exercise is advisable. Avoid tight sports bras, which many exercising, breastfeeding mothers associate with aggravating mastitis (areas of inflammation in the breast milk ducts).

Experienced runners benefit by focusing on PF and core exercises before attempting running. Leaking with running indicates the pelvic floor is not coping with the impact of the foot hitting the ground, plus the intestines and pelvic organs pushing down. You may feel fine running but cannot see what is happening inside, as supporting tissues stretch due to ineffective pelvic floor support.

Leaking towards the end of a long walk or run indicates PF muscles are fatigued and require more training in their endurance and strength modes. Change from high to low impact exercise such as walking, deep water running, swimming and easy dancing, while continuing to strengthen pelvic control.

When runners resume their fitness program, I suggest they start by running for one to two minutes then walking for 10 to 15 minutes, and repeating this pattern while slowly increasing the running period and decreasing the walking period. Progress is guided by pelvic floor control rather than focusing on the running time. Only increase the run distance when the pelvic floor is coping at the previous level.

Don't rush back to running early postpartum as pregnancy weight gains add to stress on the PF and pelvic, hip and leg joints. Regular walking or swimming and following a low G.I. eating plan are healthy ways to lose pregnancy weight gains, while gaining core and PF stability.

Stretch to maintain muscle length but avoid stretching to increase flexibility until 16 to 20 weeks postpartum, when the effects of pregnancy hormones are minimal.

Shrink the Jellybelly Routine

The **shrink the jellybelly** exercises commence 24 to 48 hours after an uncomplicated vaginal birth. This early postpartum exercise routine improves PF muscle control to strengthen bladder and bowel sphincter closing pressure, build support for pelvic organs and to improve vaginal and orgasmic sensation.

Following caesarean section or perineal repair, start this program when you feel comfortable (usually 5–10 days). The light PF muscle contractions have a 'pumping' effect to assist removal of oedema (fluid) from the perineal area.

Initially, these exercises are done with light intensity, 2 to 3 times a day, for 5 repetitions *as you regain muscular control. Avoid becoming obsessive with PF exercises and doing too many repetitions, as the PF muscles have undergone the equivalent of a marathon during pregnancy and birth.*

1. Tall Posture

To help your body quickly recover a strong aligned posture, repeat the posture exercises regularly until a tall, controlled posture becomes second nature.

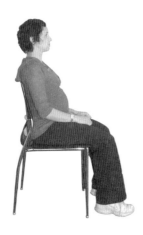

Sit in a straight-backed chair with knees comfortably apart and both feet on the ground. Position your body weight down through the sitting bones and the pubic bone in front. Sit on a pillow if stitches are uncomfortable.

Grow tall through the crown and feel lengthening through the back of your neck.

Hold this position and breathe by opening the base of the ribs. Place a pillow behind for back support, when required. When your low back softens into a slumped position, repeat this tall posture to engage pelvic floor, core and spinal muscles.

Avoid constantly lifting the sternum up to increase the lumbar curve, as this action promotes spinal muscle overactivity.

Stand with feet shoulder width apart, arms by your side, and lift up the inner arches of your feet. Grow tall through the crown as you breathe out and feel light tension as PF and core muscles switch on. Hold this position and breathe with side rib expansion. Draw up the PF with abdominal tension above the pubic bone on the out breath, using a slow, lifting action.

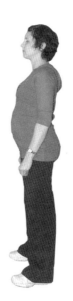

Practise *spinal lengthening* to relearn tall posture and keep the PF and core muscles active. Another great side effect of good posture is the feeling of self-confidence. When you bend, remember to keep the 'line' between the pubic bone and sternum long, and avoid curling the trunk (review this action on page 38).

2. Breathe Out to Lift

Normally the diaphragm descends internally on the in-breath but an enlarged uterus prevents the usual diaphragmatic descent. This exercise restores diaphragmatic movement and teaches the pattern of pelvic floor lifting on expiration.

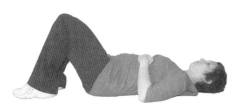

Lie on your back with both knees bent and apart. Place both hands on the lower ribs and tummy. When you breathe in, feel the breath open the ribs and abdomen, then blow out slowly though pursed lips. Practice 5 slow breaths to relearn rib-opening, diaphragmatic breathing.

On the next out breath, gently lift the PF muscles inwards (without flattening the spine onto the bed). Hold the lift for 5 seconds while breathing. Relax and repeat PF muscle lifting (on the out-breath) 5 times.

3. Pelvic Floor Lift

Imagery assists in tightening PF muscles. Imagine you are drawing a tampon in vaginally or tightening to stop passing urine. Start lying on your back, change to side lying, tall forward sitting, kneeling with head down and leaning forward over a chair with bottom out behind (knees soft).

Breathe in with rib opening; blow out slowly as you lift PF muscles. Hold for 5 seconds and repeat 5 times. Progress the hold to 10 seconds and repetitions to 10 over the next week. Refer back to page 17 for specific PF muscle exercise training.

4. Pelvic Moves

This exercise combines PF lifting with easy pelvic movement to improve control of the inner pelvic muscular corset.

Start in kneeling, in the head down, bottom up position, then in standing with bottom out as you lean onto the back of a chair or bench.

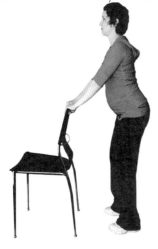

Imagine you are holding a pencil in your vagina as you slowly draw a circle with your pencil. Reverse directions and draw smaller then larger circles and figure 8's. Try to hip circle without moving the upper body.

Repeat 10 times in each direction but relax your PF to release the pencil after the exercise is finished!

5. Hissy Lift

This exercise lifts the pelvic floor with the core and all abdominal muscles. Sit tall and push both hands firmly into the sides of your waist.

Stay tall, breathe out with a long 'hissing' sound and feel your waist widen out under your hands. Relax and try again, but this time, lift your PF *first* before you get hissy.

Lift and hiss for 5 seconds, relax for 5 seconds and repeat this action 5 times, gradually lifting your floor higher with stronger hissing over the next few weeks. Use this same action with coughing, sneezing or before lifting. If the floor pushes down with the hissing action, stop the exercise and consult a women's health physiotherapist.

Stand in front of a mirror and repeat the hissy lift in your bra and undies to watch how this action shortens and tightens all abdominal muscles together.

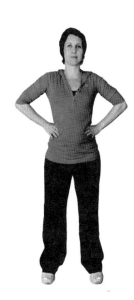

Practise this action so it becomes automatic with lifting baby or sneezing. The emphasis here is on lifting the PF muscles first–keep on lifting as you hiss. Relax muscles in between the exercises.

Warning: PF muscles tire more quickly after childbirth. The relaxation phase after each five repetitions is an essential part of this routine.

Avoid doing too many repetitions and causing muscle fatigue, aching or spasm.

6. Clam Up

The clam exercises are done slowly and then repeated with a cushion between the knees to increase PF muscle lifting. Lie on your side (hips and shoulders lined up) with both knees bent and *ankles together*. Keep the pelvis stable (don't roll back) while slowly lifting one knee up and then lowering with control. Repeat 5–10 times each side.

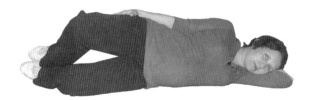

The next step is to bring knees together and squeeze a cushion (or soft ball) *lightly* for 10 seconds, breathing easily, and then relaxing for 5 seconds. Repeat 5 times.

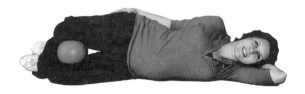

A further step is squeezing the cushion or ball again, pulsing the squeeze for 5–8 repetitions before relaxing. The emphasis is on using light squeezes to *help the pelvic floor lift higher internally* (not how hard you can squeeze).

Plan: Start with the first 4 exercises for a week, repeating them twice, then 3 times a day. The following week, add the final 2 exercises, depending on PF and abdominal comfort.

Continue these exercises for 2–4 weeks before progressing to the Train It exercises on page 163. Add the 'kneel and point' and 'hip bridging' exercises initially and each week add another 1–2 exercises. Stop any exercise that causes discomfort or pain.

Table 2. Shrink The Jellybelly Record Sheet

Week	1	2	3	4
Tall Posture				
Breathe & Lift				
Pelvic Floor Lift				
Pelvic Moves				
Hissy Lift				
Clam Up				

Instructions

Place a tick in the box each time you do the exercise during the week. Aim for at least 4 or 5 ticks in each box for four consecutive weeks to prepare for the Train It exercises.

Stretches

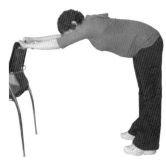

Stretch daily to release spinal muscle tension. Avoid deep stretches for 12 to 16 weeks postpartum.

Hold stretches for 20–30 seconds for 2 repetitions and breathe slowly.

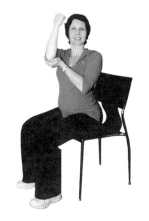
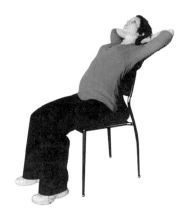

Stretches

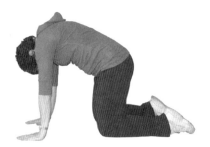
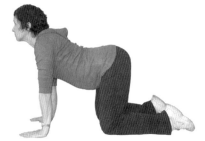

Train It Exercises

1. Hip Bridge

Lie on your back with knees bent. Breathe out, lift the PF muscles and push through heels to lift hips off the floor. Hold and breathe for 10 seconds. Lower slowly, with control, and repeat 5–10 times. Wear a support garment if you have a DRA.

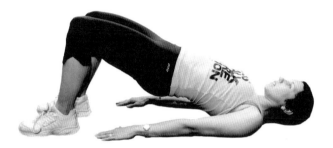

2. Arm—Leg Extension

Start on hands and knees; extend one arm and opposite leg. Hold and breathe for 10 seconds. Repeat 5 holds each side. Progress difficulty by maintaining a straight spine and bring the opposite knee and elbow towards each other. Repeat 10 times each side.

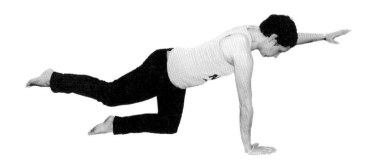

3. Sitting Control

Repeat in front of a mirror to monitor posture. Sit tall and lift the PF; take one foot off the floor. Hold and breathe for 10 seconds. Alternate left and right foot lifts for 5 to 10 repetitions. Progress by adding slow double or alternate arm lifts during the 10 second hold.

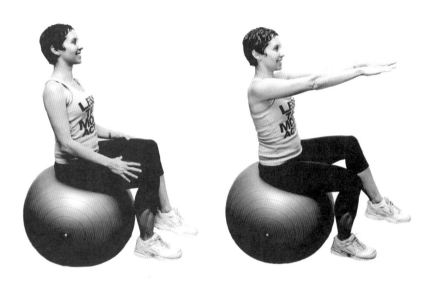

4. One Leg Balance

Stand on one leg and grow tall. Lift the PF and stay balanced as you raise the other leg to 90 degrees at the hip. Lengthen up through the supporting hip and leg, hold and breathe for 10 seconds. Repeat 5 times on each leg.

Progress by adding double or alternate arm lifts during the balance phase.

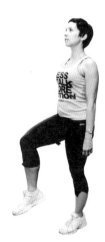

5. Stationary Running

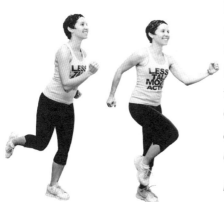

In a tall, one-leg balance stance, move your free leg in a forward/backward running action, keeping arms tucked against the body and PF muscles lifted. Only the raised leg moves—the other stays still. Repeat for 40 to 60 seconds.

Movement should be slow and controlled, concentrating on balance and smoothness. Keep the supporting leg slightly bent and stay tall. Once confident with the leg action, add the running arm action—right leg forward with left arm forward.

6. Reach and Lift

Stand on one leg with other leg to the side, just touching the floor for balance. Raise the same-side arm overhead.

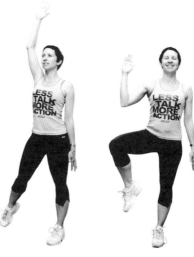

Grow tall on the supporting leg; bring your knee and elbow together.

Repeat slowly 10 times before changing sides.

7. Seated Row

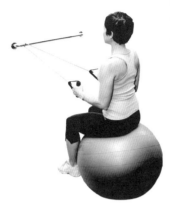

Sit on a ball or a chair, facing towards the anchor point of the stretch band. Stay tall, breathe out and lift the PF as you slowly pull elbows back. Control the PF as arms re-extend, then relax.

Do 5 to 10 repetitions. Use a lighter stretch band to learn control.

8. Standing Arm Draw

With stretch band exercises:

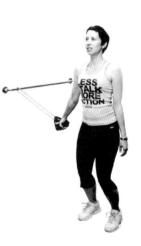

- Retain 'soft' knees. Lift the pelvic floor as you breathe out and pull the band in a slow, smooth action.
- If you lose pelvic floor lift, the resistance is too strong; use a lighter band. Do 5 to 10 repetitions.

9. Ball Squat

Place the ball behind your lower back, against the wall, feet forward and apart.

Keep pressure on the ball, squat down, letting the ball roll down the wall.

Breathe out, lift the PF and push back up through your heels. Repeat 10 times.

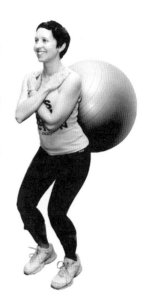

10. Balance, Lean, Pick Up

Stand on one leg; keep a straight back and balance as you bend the hip and knee to pick up an object. Repeat 3 to 5 times.

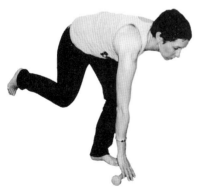

If getting to the floor is too challenging, start by placing the object on a chair or coffee table. As control improves, place the object on progressively lower surfaces.

This is not a suitable exercise after 20 weeks, or if pregnancy or postpartum pelvic girdle pain is present.

Return To Exercise

Key Points

- Don't despair if your tummy is soft and floppy as all abdominal muscles stretch to their outer range during pregnancy, but they shrink back with commitment to suitable exercises.
- Training inner muscles *first*—to recover strength and coordination is the number one priority *before* starting any aerobic, fitness or gym program.
- Challenging abdominal exercise in the first 6 months postpartum may overwhelm the smaller PF muscles. Avoid curl up and plank type exercises that isolate abdominals.
- Walk for 30 to 45 minutes most days. Adopt the tall posture when pushing the baby buggy or carrying baby in a sling.
- Wear a support garment for 4–6 weeks to control posture, support pelvic joints and compress pelvic organs.
- Delay returning to more challenging physical activity for 6 to 12 months following caesarean birth, third and fourth degree perineal tears, infection and further surgery, prolonged second stage with interventions, rectus diastasis separation, unresolved PGP, coccyx damage, prolapse and incontinence.
- Running is not suitable as an early activity due to the stress on joints and the pelvic floor.
- Eat generous servings of fruit, vegetables and lean protein rather than high GI foods such as chips, biscuits, cakes and soft drinks.
- Visit a dietician for eating guidelines if your breastfeeding appetite goes into overdrive.
- Repeat pelvic floor strength exercises 3 times a day and start the **shrink the jellybelly** program when you are comfortable after vaginal and caesarean births.

Returning to Exercise Questions for Caregivers:

SECTION 13

Birth and Postpartum Care in Other Cultures

International Birthing Practices

The birthing experience for women varies world wide from the technology led experience in some western cultures to the lack of basic maternal care in many third world countries. Following is a glimpse of birthing practices from around the world.

German women are given a Mutterpass or 'mother's passport' after visiting a gynaecologist. Any pregnancy-related conditions, chronic illnesses, and medical procedures carried out during pregnancy, plus the mother's health following the birth are recorded in the 'mother's passport'.

Pregnant women are entitled to 10 or more prenatal consultations with a midwife or doctor. German Health Insurance covers daily visits by the midwife until the baby is 10 days old and the cost of postnatal care for eight weeks following the birth. Some hospitals allow the mother to take her own midwife into the birth room.

German women can choose between an 'outpatient' birth in a hospital, birthing clinic or at the midwife or doctor's clinic. Birthing houses offer holistic, non-clinical outpatient births and antenatal care. These houses are close to hospitals for emergency care and are operated by midwives and occupational therapists.

Home births are performed with a qualified midwife who visits daily until baby is 10 days old. After this time, health insurance covers further home visits or phone consultations with a midwife, along with postnatal classes for pelvic floor strengthening.

Japanese women, influenced by centuries of tradition, give birth without painkillers, although more doctors are recommending an epidural for pain relief. Two prenatal visits with a doctor (who performs many tests) are free of charge as are childbirth classes. Japanese women, who follow older customs, wrap a white cloth around the abdomen during the fifth month of pregnancy symbolising their wish for an easy birth and visit Shinto shrines to pray for a safe pregnancy.

Small clinics provide a home like atmosphere for Japanese women to birth, where the midwives encourage traditional birthing styles with labouring done on Tatami matting. The idea of the father being present at the birth is often viewed as a novelty. When birthing in a hospital, women are expected to stay for five days after a vaginal birth and 10 days after a caesarean birth. New mothers often stay with their baby at her parents' home and remain in bed with baby for 21 days. Friends join the family in greeting the new baby and eat Osekihan, a celebratory dish of red beans with red rice.

Postnatal belly binding, called Haramaki, is common in Japan. It claims to reverse flabby tummies with correct posture and support.

Brazilian women frequently request and are encouraged by their doctors to have a caesarean birth. According to the International Caesarean Awareness Network, the overall rate of caesarean births in Brazil is 40 percent and up to 70 percent in some private hospitals. A Brazilian colleague told me she was constantly asked to explain why she chose to birth vaginally rather than by caesarean section. She also spoke of a caesarean rate in some private hospitals of 90 percent. Home and water births are not common and it is difficult to find a facility or obstetrician to support these births.

The mother stays in hospital for up to three days after giving birth, and longer following a caesarean birth. Maternity hospitals run pre- and postnatal care classes. Pregnant women are given priority treatment and made to feel special. Once mother and baby leave the hospital, visitors bring presents for the baby and receive a small gift in return.

In **France,** pregnant women receive a pass, the Carnet de Santé Maternité, which gives them the right to go to the front of a queue or obtain a seat on public transport. Pregnant women are obliged to have seven prenatal examinations. They usually birth in a maternity hospital with a midwife, staying in hospital for around three days.

Home births are not common in France for various administrative and insurance reasons and fear of prosecution for birth assistants if something goes wrong. Despite this, home births are now requested more often.

Local healthcare centres provide postnatal checks, and advice with breastfeeding and nutrition. French women are the envy of many mothers worldwide as they receive up to 10 free postnatal physiotherapy sessions to restore their PF function. Vive la France!

In **China**, nearly half of all pregnant women choose a caesarean birth, according to a report from the World Health Organization (WHO recommends caesarean birth rates should be no higher than 15 per cent).

During a woman's first birth, her mother attends and although the baby's father is not present, he is expected to give the baby its first bath. Traditionally, Chinese women laboured in an armchair or futon and squatted to birth.

The mother of the pregnant woman sends her daughter a package, tsue shen ('hastening delivery'), which contains a white cloth, in which to wrap the baby. The new mother is expected to stay in bed and avoid heavy work for 30 days (the sitting month) after baby is born.

In **Holland** the doctor only intervenes if complications arise in labour or if the mother is 'high risk' and refers most pregnant mothers to a local midwife. The Dutch believe pregnant women should not be treated as patients because having a baby is not a medical condition.

Women can decide if they want to birth at home or in a hospital. Typically, 30 per cent of Dutch births take place at home (compared with over 90 per cent of births in the U.S. taking place in a hospital environment). The Health Insurer sends a Kraampakket (home birthing box) containing all the items needed for a home birth.

When a hospital birth is chosen, the midwife visits the labouring mother in her home and advises on the best time to go to hospital. Dutch women typically expect to give birth vaginally without pain medication (only 10 per cent of Dutch women use pain relief). Instead, the emphasis is on relaxation and breathing techniques in prenatal yoga classes. Engaging a Doula for support and guidance during and after labour is becoming more popular.

Medical insurance funds the Kraamzorg service, which provides a nurse to visit the mother in her home for a week. The nurse offers advice on postnatal care, breastfeeding and helps to care for other children. Some even help with the cooking!

In **Spain** women give birth at state owned social security hospitals or private clinics. Prenatal examinations are done by a midwife or doctor, then regularly throughout the pregnancy. Some clinics provide prenatal classes to prepare the mother (and father) for labour.

Women expect to stay in hospital for 48 hours following a vaginal birth and up to five days following a caesarean birth. Home births are not generally available in Spain and postnatal care is limited.

In **Russia**, home births aided by only a midwife or doctor have gained popularity over the past 20 years due in part to financial savings and concerns about how the mother may be treated in a maternity ward. State-owned maternity hospitals have sections for paying and non-paying patients, or where fathers stay with their family. A few maternity hospitals are setting up homebirth centers (Domashniye Rody) with home-like rooms for women wanting to avoid the typical hospital experience.

Currently caesarean births account for 16 to 20 per cent of births in Moscow's maternity hospitals, requiring a six-day hospital stay, instead of the usual four days following a vaginal birth.

It is Russian policy for women who have attended prenatal classes and checkups for 12 weeks, to receive a 'childbirth certificate', which entitles them to 2,000 rubles for prenatal care and 5,000 rubles towards birth costs. These payments are due for an upward revision along with the introduction of monthly payments for educational expenses and home improvements, accessible only after the child turns three years old.

For **Swedish** women, childbirth is a normal event managed with minimal intervention. A specialist midwife or Barnmorskor monitors pregnancy, childbirth and postnatal care. An obstetrician is only consulted if the midwife becomes aware of complications or is concerned for the health of the mother and baby.

Expectant parents are encouraged to attend pre- and postnatal classes. Childbirth takes place in a birthing unit, often with a doula for assistance. The father is encouraged to attend the birth, with the midwife birthing the baby, only calling the obstetrician if complications arise. Caesarean section on-demand is not encouraged in Sweden.

Folllowing birth, mother and baby are taken to a 'patient' hotel for 48 hours, which is staffed by a midwife and nurse assistants. The father is also welcome to stay. Planned home and water births are not encouraged in Sweden. Midwives visit the new mother at home if she is not coping and requires more care and support.

The practise of abdominal binding in the post natal period is widely practised and reported in the **Hmong, Japanese, Mayan, African, Filipina, Malaysian, Indonesian and Singaporean** cultures. The binding is done to bring the mother's abdomen back to its normal shape and improve her posture. Binding is promoted as being more effective when combined with abdominal massage. The western equivalent to abdominal binding is a support garment or girdle.

Pregnant women in **third world countries** experience a high rate of child and maternal deaths and birth injuries through lack of trained local birth attendants. Reports from the UNFPA (United Nations Population Fund) show a soaring rate of maternal deaths in the Solomon Islands, Laos, East Timor, Indonesia and Papua New Guinea due to the lack of skilled birth attendants and low spending on maternal health.

The ICS (International Continence Society) reports the risk of dying in pregnancy or labour for African women to be one in 12. They state: 'For every woman who dies in labour in the developing world, many more find their lives destroyed by terrible injuries because of untreated obstructed labour. The developed world is now only becoming aware of the devastation to women's lives, largely because women in the developing world have no voice in the international community'.

The Addis Ababa Fistula Hospital was founded by Dr Catherine Hamlin AC and her late husband, Dr Reg Hamlin OBE, and is dedicated to the treatment and care of women who suffer horrendous childbirth injuries, known as obstetric fistula.

Dr Hamlin reports 'Obstetric fistula is caused by prolonged obstructed labour when a woman will spend days in labour without any medical help or pain relief. If she survives this ordeal, she will give birth to a stillborn child and her internal injuries will cause urinary and sometimes, faecal incontinence. A woman like this will spend the rest of her life a destitute outcast unless she can get to the Addis Ababa Fistula Hospital or one of its outreach centres.'

The Addis Ababa Fistula Hospital is committed to the UN Millennium Development Goals and particularly those directed towards improving maternal health, reducing infant mortality and empowering women. It has established the Hamlin College of Midwives to train young Ethiopian women as midwives to work in the countryside amongst women who presently have little or no access to medical help during their pregnancy and labour. The mission of the Hamlin College of Midwives is to have a midwife in every Ethiopian village.

The following story concerns a young woman who visited me for pelvic floor advice following the birth of her first child. Lottie experienced depression, isolation and anger after her first traumatic birth in a large, busy city hospital in Australia. To birth her second baby she decided to return to her grandmother's home in Indonesia.

I was fascinated as she related her birth experience at her grand-mother's home. At five months, a local midwife commenced regular full body massage along with mixing special pregnancy herb teas for Lottie. During her seventh month, the midwife started abdominal massage to correct the baby's uterine position.

When labour began, Lottie walked and sat as her midwife used firm back and abdominal massage to help control strong contractions. The room was quiet with only her grandmother and midwife present. She didn't remember the length of her labour, just that is was calm and unhurried.

After her daughter was born, Lottie was visited daily by her midwife who prepared a therapeutic bath, made herb tea to promote breast milk production, performed a full body massage, and wrapped her abdomen.

Lottie was encouraged to move around the house and walk regularly but did not cook or clean until she stopped bleeding. The daily ritual with her midwife continued for 40 days, after which Lottie assured me she felt emotionally and physically strong to return home to her busy life in Australia (and fitted easily into her jeans)!

Lottie's vastly different experience between her two births stayed etched in my memory. Her story is just one that highlights the importance of educating, listening to, nuturing and protecting women during and after their time of miraculous creation.

Vaginal birth without intervention is currently recognised as the safest way to birth for both mother and baby (for low risk women).

Women's perceptions of their birth experiences remain with them for life. I sincerely hope the information in this book plays a role in allowing you to retain lifetime memories of joy and fulfillment associated with your births.

SECTION 14

Beyond Birth

A Healthy Pelvic Floor For Life

With the joy of motherhood comes possibly the busiest time of life as you raise children, pursue careers, attend children's school and sporting events and organise family celebrations. Making time to restore and maintain ongoing dynamic pelvic stability may not register on your list of priorities. But wait, stay with me a little longer. The years ahead are filled with the physical loading of lifting heavy children, moving house and attacking gardens, caring for ageing parents, enjoying family adventure holidays and trying new exercise programs. Then comes the peri- and menopausal years when activity often slows and maybe new signs of pelvic floor issues appear.

The main focus of Hold It Mama has been the pelvic floor during pregnancy and birth; yet many other factors and habits throughout your life greatly influence pelvic floor function. This section contains advice related to ongoing pelvic health throughout life.

Occasionally I hear the response 'what's there to know about my bladder and bowel? I just go to the toilet and that's that'! To improve or maintain smooth elimination, it's never too late to learn more about these often ignored organs. Keep your bladder happy by

- Giving artificial sweeteners a wide berth to avoid urgency. (Recent research shows diet soda increases the risk of stroke, myocardial infarct or vascular death by 61 per cent in regular users compared with those who drink no diet soda).
- Sit tall with a relaxed abdomen when voiding to prevent the habit of bearing down internally to empty (a cause of urgency).

Relaxing the abdominal wall and pelvic floor cues the sphincters to relax and then the bladder muscles contract to empty urine.

- Keeping your PC in top working order as this little muscle controls the sphincters preventing urine loss and also shuts down the urgency sensation.
- Checking your emptying habits – up to 5 or 6 voids a day and once at night is considered normal. Putting off toilet visits in a busy working situation over distends bladder walls, which may lead to less responsive bladder muscles. Avoid emptying until you have at least 250mls of stored urine.

The bowel is a barometer for the health of your body. Keep it happily emptying by

- Creating meals with fruit, vegetables, legumes and whole grains to gain fibre and friendly bacteria for a healthy bowel. Consistently eating low or no fibre foods causes constipation and straining. Regularly passing a 'silicone coated sausage' is the mark of a healthy bowel.
- Adopting low glycaemic eating habits. Regularly eating high glycaemic foods creates an acidic cellular environment, which promotes inflammation and is associated with bladder and bowel dysfunction.
- Taking time to sit and relax in a forward lean position promotes full bowel emptying.
- Speaking with bowel and nutrition specialists if irritable bowel symptoms, food intolerances or pain alter your regular emptying pattern.

Exercise to retain healthy pelvic floor muscles by

- Pursuing pelvic friendly exercise with dance (belly, jazz, free form and latin), tai chi, yoga and low-level aerobics. Exercising with movement and controlled posture suits the female body rather than focusing on isolating movement (sit ups) and prolonged trunk bracing (plank holds).

- Enjoy exercise you plan to continue throughout life – walking, golf, dance, yoga and swimming. Forget about 'punishing routines' as they are potentially pelvic floor damaging and not sustainable. Regular exercise should bring a heightened sense of wellbeing and improved health.

- Becoming a stickler for controlling posture whether you are stationary or active. Controlling posture keeps core muscles active in their endurance mode to counteract wear and tear on joints.

- Incorporating specific pelvic floor exercises into daily exercises or activities. Lift your pelvic floor before picking up an object or increase pelvic floor lifting with hip liberating, belly dancing moves.

- To flatten your stomach or switch on abdominals with exercise, lift from the pelvic floor first. Regularly take deep breaths to open the base of your ribs to keep the diaphragm and pelvic floor working in coordinated harmony.

Protect against prolapse by

- Being realistic about how much you can safely lift. You are not invincible and most women are not suited to labouring work or helping to carry the fridge! Train your children to climb up into their car seats and to ask for a sitting down cuddle. Having a vagina creates a space into which pelvic organs may potentially descend when the pelvic floor muscles are continually overpowered by internal pressure rises.

- Ignoring the person beside you in an exercise class – tune into how your body responds to or controls an exercise. If you cannot maintain the small inward low back curve or your abdomen and pelvic floor bulge, stop the activity and try an easier option.

- Using the 'knack' (page 21) to lift from underneath before the everyday actions of lifting, sneezing, pushing and pulling.

- Sitting down to cough if you have the flu or an ongoing chest infection. Use hand pressure up over your perineum to augment the 'knack' lifting action. Sure, it's a challenge to do this walking through town, so in a public situation drop your purse and squat down with your perineum pressed on the back of one ankle (the other foot is flat).

- Keeping poos soft (as in the silicone sausage) reduces the risk of pelvic organ prolapse. With a back wall prolapse, placing thumb pressure against the back vaginal wall gives support to help the bowel empty without straining. Pelvic floor muscle strengthening improves overall organ support, may reduce a front wall prolapse and controls (does not reduce) a back wall prolapse.

Orgasm (with or without a partner) provides a natural work out for pelvic muscles and releases pleasurable hormones (orgasm releases oxytocin, the 'love hormone' that bonds partners together). Dr Christiane Northrup writes about nitric oxide, the 'pleasure hormone', which is released with orgasm or other joyous experiences. This gas is released from blood vessel walls and increases the production of neurotransmitters that improve mood and wellbeing.

Women experience longer orgasms than men, which is great news for working out your pelvic floor muscles. Contractions begin in the uterus, fallopian tubes, rectum and pelvic floor muscles with repeated contractions. The vagina operates best during intercourse with lubrication from vascular engorgement and gland secretions. Augment lubrication when needed (postpartum, menopause, post surgery or radiation) to reduce discomfort and improve pleasure.

Take time throughout life to experience orgasmic joy, revel in eating the delights nature produces and enjoy empowering exercise and share these activities with family and friends (mostly the eating and exercise).

Finally dear readers, think of your pelvic floor muscles as the Queen of your core muscles. Continue to keep the Queen happily reigning throughout your life by:

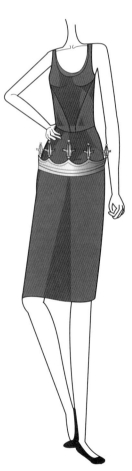

- Becoming her biggest admirer and supporter for the myriad of roles she coordinates in your body.
- Preparing for and respecting her role in birth and guiding her back to her former self to reign with dynamic stability.
- Tall posture to keep her regally 'switched on'.
- Using the 'knack' to lift and support her before activity.
- Never overpowering her with heavy lifting.
- Regular exercises to keep her strong and in control to prevent disruption and upheaval throughout her life.
- Avoiding over challenging exercises that may overwhelm and topple her reigning status.
- Letting her rest and relax between exercises to prevent her from becoming uptight.

- Controlling your waistline so she does not feel the 'weight of the world' upon her.
- Eating fibre rich foods and drinking enough water to avoid her straining with elimination.
- Keeping her happy with dance, yoga, tai chi and exercise involving the mind/body connection.
- Adoring and honouring her with frequent pleasure for a lifetime of wellbeing.

Pelvic Floor Assessment Chart

Complete the following responses and take the completed chart to your doctor if 'yes' answers are recorded.

Bladder	No	Yes
Do you lose urine with sneezing or exercising?		
Does urgency cause frequent voiding?		
Do you lose urine due to sudden urgency?		
Do you empty more than 6 times daily?		
At night, do you get up more than once to empty?		
Do you lose urine at night in bed?		
Have you stopped exercising due to urine loss?		
Is urine loss affecting your quality of life?		
Bowel		
Does your bowel empty more than 3 times per day?		
Does your bowel empty less than twice per week?		
Do you have difficulty controlling wind?		
Do you occasionally lose bowel matter?		
Do you strain to empty your bowel?		
Do you have haemorrhoids or anal fissures?		
Is it difficult to fully empty your bowel?		
Intimacy		
Do you have pain with intercourse?		
Has vaginal sensation with intercourse diminished?		
Is your orgasm less intense?		
Prolapse		
Does your pelvic floor feel 'heavier' at end of day?		
Do you have a bulge at your vaginal entrance?		
Do you experience abdominal, vaginal or back pain?		
Count the total 'Yes' answers:		

48 Hour Bladder Chart

Date	Time	Vol (ml)	Pad Status	Pad Change	Fluid Intake
12 Sep	6.05am	550	N/A	N/A	300ml water
	9.45am	240	Damp	YES	250ml coffee
Total Output			**Total Intake**		

Pad Status: dry/damp/wet/soaked
Pad Change: Did you change pad? Yes or No (N/A if not using pads)
Fluid Intake – list all consumed

7 Day Bowel Chart

Date	Time	Urgency	Loss type	Strain to open	Pain	Blood	Consistency & shape
4 Jun	2pm	No	W	Yes	rectum	Yes	Hard, lumpy
7 Jun	8am	Yes	L	No	No	No	Loose, pebbles

Urgency Feeling of marked urgency? Yes / No
Loss Involuntary loss of **S**olid, **L**iquid, **M**ucous or **W**ind – or **N**one
Strain Difficulty emptying / manual assistance – Yes / No

Pain Yes / No – if yes, note location
Bleeding Yes / No
Consistency eg: hard/loose/watery
Shape eg: sausage/pebbles/lumpy

SECTION 15

Information and References

Internet Resources

Midwives

midwives.org.au
australiansocietyofindependentmidwives.com
homebirthaustralia.org
maternitycoalition.org.au
midwife.org.nz

Continence Organisations

continence.org.au
continence.org.nz

Physiotherapy Associations

physiotherapy.asn.au
physiotherapy.org.nz

Obstetricians and Gynaecologists

ranzcog.edu.au

Constipation

cssa.org.au/content/4/37onstipation
gesa.org.au/leaflets/constipation.cfm

Collagen Weakness/Hypermobile Joints

hypermobility.org

The Bellybra

bellybra.com

Recovery Shorts

recoveryshorts.com.au

Pelvic Pain

pelvicpain.org

pelvicpartnership.org.uk

sexwithoutpain.com

vaginismus.com

Interstitial Cystitis

ic-network.com

Pelvic Girdle Pain / Pelvic Instability

pelvicgirdlepain.com/pelvic-girdle-pain.htm

Exercise Guidelines During Pregnancy

acog.org/publications/patient_education/bp119.cfm

http://sma.org.au/wp-content/uploads/2009/05/torode.pdf

acog.org/publications/patient_education/bp119.cfm

Pink Kits

thepinkkit.com

Office Ergonomics

ergonomics.com.au

Belly Dance for Pregnancy and Birth DVD

bellydanceforbirth.com

Birth Rights

mybirth.com.au

childbirthconnection.org

Caesarean Birth

caesarean.org.uk

canaustralia.net

postoppain.org

Caesarean Scars Silicone scar sheets

rejuveness.com

pharmacyonline.com.au

Birth Information For Couples

birth.com.au

activebirthcentre.com

birthingfromwithin.com

Books:

Active Birth Books

Birthing From Within, Pam England

The Water Birth Book. Janet Balaskas

Foetal Monitoring

childbirth.org/articles/efmfaq.html

Epidurals

americanpregnancy.org/labornbirth/epidural.html

womenshealthmatters.ca/centres/pregnancy/childbirth/epidural.
html

Episiotomy

mayoclinic.com/health/episiotomy/HO00064

Rupture of the Membranes

midwife.org.nz/index.cfm/3,108,559/arm-consensus-statement-
2008-final.pdf

Vaginal Pessary for Prolapse

thewomens.org.au/Vaginalpessaryforprolapse

International Caesarean Awareness Network

ican-online.org

Postnatal Depression

panda.org.au

beyondblue.org.au

blackdoginstitute.org.au

Breastfeeding

breastfeeding.asn.au

VBAC Support

canaustralia.net

cares-sa.org.au

birthrites.org

Glycemic Index Foundation newsletter

ginews.blogspot.com

The Hamlin Fistula Organisation

hamlinfistula.org.au

Vaginal Exercisers

pelvicfloorexercise.com.au

incostress.com

Further Reading

Balaskas J (2004). The Water Birth Book. Thorsons.

Buckley SJ. (2009). Gentle Birth, Gentle Mothering. A Doctor's guide to natural childbirth and gentle early parenting choices. Celestial Arts.

Chippington-Derrick D. (2005). Caesarean Birth: Your questions asnwered. NCT Publishers.

England P, Horowitz R. (1998). Birthing from Within: An Extra-Ordinary Guide to Childbirth Preparation. Partera Press.

Fahri D. (1996). The Breathing Book, Good health and vitality through essential breath work. Owl Books, Henry Holt and company, New York.

Herrera I (2009). Ending Female Pain. Duplex Publishing New York

King R (2010). Where Did My Libido Go? Random House Australia.

Kitzinger S. The new pregnancy and childbirth. Dorling Kindersley.

Mayo Clinic (2004). Mayo Clinic Guide to a Healthy Pregnancy. Harper Paperbacks.

Northrup C. (2010). Women's Bodies, Women's Wisdom (Revised Edition): Creating Physical and Emotional Health and Healing. Bantam.

O'Dwyer M. (2010). Hold It Sister: (Revised edition):The Confident Girl's Guide To a Leak-Free Life. Redsok.

Price C, Robinson S. (2010). Birth: Conceiving, Nurturing And Giving Birth To Your Baby. Macmillan.

Sears W, Sears M. (1994). The Birth Book: Everything you need to know to have a safe and satisfying birth. Little, Brown & Company.

Trotter S. (2004). Breastfeeding: The essential Guide. Trotters Independent Publishing.

Wise D, Anderson R. (2008) 5th edition. A headache in the pelvis: A new understanding for chronic pelvic pain syndromes. National centre for pelvic pain research. Occidental California.

References

Section 1. The Pelvic Floor

Sapsford R, Hodges P, Richardson C. Activation of the abdominal muscles in a normal response to contraction of the pelvic floor muscles. Conference abstract p 117. ISC 1997. Yokohama.

Kiff E, Barnes P, Swash M. Evidence of pudendal neuropathy in patients with perineal descent and chronic straining at stool Gut 1984 25:1279-1282

Subak LL. Weight loss to treat urinary incontinence in overweight and obese women. NEJM 2009.Vol 360:481-490(5).

Fynes M. Effect of pregnancy and delivery on posterior vaginal compartment. ISC proceedings 2003, Florence.

Salvesen K, Mørkved S. Randomised controlled trial of pelvic floor muscle training during pregnancy. BMJ. 2004 August 14; 329(7462): 378–380.doi: 10.1136/bmj.38163.724306.3A

Wesnes SL, Hunskaar S, Bo K, and Rortveit G. Urinary Incontinence and Weight Change During Pregnancy and Postpartum: A Cohort Study. Am J Epidemiol. 2010 November 1; 172(9): 1034–1044.

O'Sullivan P, Twomey L, Allison G: Altered patterns of abdominal muscle activation in chronic back pain patients. Aust J Physio 43(2):91-98, 1997

Jack G, Kikolova G, Vilain E, Raz S, Rodriguez L, Familial transmission of genitovaginal prolapse. Int Urogyn J 2006. Vol 17(5):498-501

Norton PA, Baker JE, Sharp HC, Warenski JC. Genitourinary prolapse and joint hypermobility in women. Obstet Gynecol. 1995 Feb;85(2):225-8.

Sampsele C, Miller J, Mims B, Delancey J, Ashton-Miller J, Antonakos C. Effect of pelvic floor muscle exercise on transient incontinence during pregnancy and after birth. O&G 1998;91(3):406-412

Eason E, Labrecque M, Marcoux S, Mondor M. Effects of carrying a pregnancy and method of delivery on urinary incontinence: a prospective cohort study. BMC Preg Child 2004;4:4.

Nixon G, Glazner J, Martin T, Sawyer S. Urinary incontinence in female adolescents after cystic fibrosis. Pediatrics 2002;110;2: e22

Hunskaars S, A systematic review of overweight and obesity as risk factors and targets for clinical intervention for urinary incontinence in women. Neurourol Urodyn 2008;28(8):749-757

Maserejian N, Giovannucci E, McVary K, McGrotherand C, McKinlay J.Dietary Macronutrient and Energy Intake and Urinary Incontinence in Women. Am. J. Epidemiol. (2010) 171 (10): 1116-1125.

Smith MD, Russell A, Hodges PW (2008) Is there a relationship between parity, pregnancy, back pain and incontinence? International Urogynecology Journal and Pelvic Floor Dysfunction 19: 205–211.

Stapleton DB, MacLennan AH, Kristiansson P (2002) The prevalence of recalled lower back pain during and after pregnancy: a South Australian population survey. Australian and New Zealand Journal of Obstetrics and Gynaecology 42:Issue 5: 482–485.

Section 2: Pregnancy

Bo, K. (2009). Does pelvic floor muscle training prevent and treat urinary and fecal incontinence in pregnancy? Nat Clin Pract Urol, 6(3), 122-123.

Hay-Smith J, Morkved S, Fairbrother K, Herbison G. Pelvic floor muscle training for prevention and treatment of urinary and faecal incontinence in ante natal and post natal women. Evid Based Med. 2009;14(2):53

Morkved S, Bo K, Schei B, Salvesen KA. Pelvic floor muscle training during pregnancy to prevent urinary incontinence: A single-blind randomized controlled trial. O&G. 2003. 101: 313-319.

Jack G, Kikolova G, Vilain E, Ras S, Rodriguez L. Familial transmission of genitovaginal prolapse. Int Urogyn 2006;17(5):498-501

Norton P. Pelvic floor disorders:the role of fascia and ligaments. Clin Obstst Gynaec 1993;36:926-938

Pool-Goudzwaard AL, Slieker ten Hove MC, Vierhout ME, Mulder PH, Pool JJ, Snijders CJ, et al. Relations between pregnancy-related low back pain, pelvic floor activity and pelvic floor dysfunction. Int.U.J.Pelvic Floor Dys. 2005;16(6):468-474.

Albert HB, Godskesen M, Korsholm L, Westergaard JG. Risk factors in developing pregnancy-related pelvic girdle pain. Acta Obstet.Gynecol.Scand. 2006;85(5):539-544.

Larsen E, Wilken-Jensen C, Hansen A, Jensen D, Johansen S, Minck H, et al. Symptom-giving pelvic girdle relaxation in pregnancy. I: Prevalence and risk factors. Acta Obstet.Gynecol.Scand. 1999 Feb;78(2):105-110.

Vleeming A, Albert H, Ostgaard H, Sturesson B, Stuge B. European guidelines on the diagnosis and treatment of pelvic girdle pain European Commission Research Directorate General Website 2005. backpaineurope.org/web/files/WG4_Guidelines.pdf

Hammer RL, Perkins J, Parr R. Exercise during the childbearing year. J Perinat Educ. 2000;9:1–14.

Vleeming A, Albert HB, Ostgaard HC, Sturesson B, Stuge B. European guidelines for the diagnosis and treatment of pelvic girdle pain. Eur.Spine J. 2008 Jun;17(6):794-819.

Boissonnault J, Blaschak M. Incidence of diastasis recti abdominis during the childbearing year. Physical Therapy 1988;68:1082-1086

Spitznagel T, Leong F, Van Dillen L. Prevelance of diastasis recti Abdominis in a urogynaelogical population. Int Urogyn J. 2007Vol 18(3):321-328.

Abramowitz L. Anal fissure and thrombosed external hemorrhoids before and after delivery. Dis Colon Rectum 2002;45:650-5.

Guyton, Hall 2005. Textbook of Medical Physiology (11 ed.) Philadelphia: Saunders. pp. 103g. ISBN 81-8147-920-3.

The Royal Australian and New Zealand College of Obstetricians and Gynaecologists. Use of prostaglandins for cervical ripening prior to the induction of labour [online]. 2009 [Cited 2010 Feb 10]. Available from: http://ranzcog.edu.au/publications/statements/C-obs22.pdf

ACOG committee opinion:exercise during pregnancy and the post partum period. ACOG Int Gynaec Obstet 2002;77:79-81

Kramer M, McDonald SW. Aerobic Exercise for Women During Pregnancy. Cochrane Database Systematic Review. 2006;(3): CD000180.

The Physical Activity Readiness Medical Examination for Pregnancy (PARmed-X for Pregnancy) csep.ca/forms.asp

Mottola M, Davenport M, Brun C, Inglis S, Charlesworth S, Sopper M. VO2 peak prediction and exercise prescription for pregnant women. Med Sci Sports Exerc. 2006;38:1389-1395.

Baciuk E, Baciuk P,Pereira R, Cecatti J, Braga A, Cavalcante S. Water aerobics in pregnancy: Cardiovascular response, labor and neonatal outcomes. Reprod Health. 2008 Nov 21;5:10.

Bø K, Fleten C, Nystad W. Effect of antenatal pelvic floor muscle training on labor and birth. Obstet Gynecol. 2009 Jun;113(6):1279-84.

Hoff Braekken I, Majida M, Engh M, Bo K. Morphological changes after pelvic floor muscle trainng measured by 3D ultrasonography:a randominised controlled trial. O&G 2011;115:317-324

Section 3: Preparing For Labour

Beckmann MM, Garrett AJ. Antenatal perineal massage for reducing perineal trauma. Cochrane Database of Systematic Reviews 2006, Issue 1. Art. No.: CD005123. DOI: 10.1002/14651858.CD005123.pub2

Parente MP, Natal Jorge RM, Mascarenhas T, Silva-Filho AL. The influence of pelvic muscle activation during vaginal delivery. O&G. 2010;115(4):804-8. PMID: 20308842

Shek K, Langer SE, Chantarasorn V, Dietz H. Does the Epi-No device prevent levator trauma? A randomised controlled trial. Ultrasound in O&G. Volume 36, Issue S1, page 93, 2010

Lawrence A, Lewis L, Hofmeyr GJ, Dowswell T, Styles C. Maternal positions and mobility during first stage labour. Cochrane Database 2009, Issue 2. Art. No.: CD003934. DOI: 10.1002/14651858.CD003934.pub2

Hofmeyr GJ, Kulier R. Hands and knees posture in late pregnancy or labour for foetal malposition (lateral or posterior). Birth. 2005; 32:235–236.

Cluett ER, Burns E. Immersion in water in labour and birth. Cochrane Database of Systematic Reviews 2009, Issue 2. Art. No.: CD000111. DOI: 10.1002/14651858.CD000111.pub3

Gupta JK, Hofmeyr GJ, Smyth R. Position in the second stage of labour for women without epidural anaesthesia. The Coch Database of Sys Rev 2004; 1. Art. No.: CD002006. DOI:10.1002/14651858.CD002006.pub2.

Dowswell T, Bedwell C, Lavender T, Neilson JP. Transcutaneous electrical nerve stimulation (TENS) for pain relief in labour. Cochrane Database of Systematic Reviews 2009, Issue 2. Art. No.: CD007214. DOI: 10.1002/14651858. CD007214.pub2

Fahy K, Hastie C, Bisits A, Marsh C, Smith L, Saxton A. Holistic physiological care compared with active management of the third stage of labour for women at low risk of postpartum haemorrhage: A cohort study. Women and Birth 23;2010:146-152

Section 4: Interventions during labour

Alfirevic Z, Devane D, Gyte GML. Continuous cardiotocography (CTG) as a form of electronic fetal monitoring (EFM) for fetal assessment during labour. Cochrane Database of Systematic Reviews 2006, Issue 3. Art. No.: CD006066. DOI: 10.1002/14651858.CD006066

Anim-Somuah M, Smyth RMD, Howell CJ. Epidural versus non-epidural or no analgesia in labour. Cochrane Database of Systematic Reviews 2005,Issue4. Art.No.:CD000331.DOI:10.1002/14651858.CD000331.pub2

Lieberman E, Davidson K, Lee-Parritz A, Shearer E (2005). Changes in fetal position during labor and their association with epidural anesthesia. Obstetrics & Gynaecology, 105(5, Part 1) 974-982

Parente M,Natal Jorge R,Mascarenhas T,Fernandes A, Martins J. The influence of an occipito-posterior malposition on the biomechanical behavior of the pelvic floor. EJOG;1: S166-S169 (May 2009)

De Tayrac R, Panel L, Masson G, Mares P. Episiotomy and prevention of pelvic floor and perineal injuries. Gyn Obst Biol Reprod 2006;35(1):1S24

Carolli G, Belizan J. Episiotomy for vaginal birth. 2001. Cochrane Database Systematic Review: CD 000081

Boulvain M, Stan CM, Irion O. Membrane sweeping for induction of labour. Cochrane Database of Systematic Reviews 2005, Issue 1. Art. No.: CD000451. DOI: 10.1002/14651858.CD000451.pub2

Meyer S, Hohlfeld P, 2001. Birth trauma: Short and long term effects of forceps delivery compared with spontaneous delivery on various pelvic floor parameters. BGOJ 107(11):1360-1370.

O'Mahony F, Hofmeyr GJ, Menon V. Choice of instruments for assisted vaginal delivery. Cochrane Database of Systematic Reviews 2010, Issue 11. Art. No.: CD005455. DOI: 10.1002/14651858.CD005455.pub2

Parente M,Natal Jorge R,Mascarenhas T,Fernandes A, Martins J. The influence of an occipito-posterior malposition on the biomechanical behavior of the pelvic floor. EJOG;1: S166-S169 (May 2009)

Electronic Medical Compendium: http://www.medicines.org.uk/EMC/
medicine/16424/SPC/Syntocinon+Ampoules+10+IU+ml/

Section 5: Birth

Smith, C., & Dahlen, H. Caring for the pregnant woman and her baby in a
changing maternity service environment: the role of acupuncture. Acupuncture
in Medicine, 2009; 27(3). 123-125.

Phumdoung S, Pool M. Music reduces sensation and distress of labour pain.
Pain Management Nursing. 2003;4(2):54-61.

Hodnett ED, Gates S, Hofmeyr GJ, Sakala C. Continuous support for women
during childbirth.Cochrane Data Syst Rev. 2003;(3):CD003766.

Caldeyro-Barcia R. The influence of maternal position on time of spontaneous
rupture of the membranes, progress of labour, and foetal head compression.
Birth Family Journal 1979b; 6:7-15.

Sakala C. Vaginal or Caesarean Birth? A Systematic Review to Determine What
is at Stake for Mothers and Babies. Childbirth Connection 2006.

Anim-Somuah M, Smyth RMD, Howell CJ. Epidural versus non-epidural or no
analgesia in labour. Cochrane Database of Systematic Reviews 2005, Issue 4.
Art. No.: CD000331. DOI: 10.1002/14651858.CD000331.pub2

Stark MA, Jones M. Advanced Preparation and Positive Labor Support Create
an Optimal Experience for Normal Birth. J Perinatal Education. 2006 ;15(2):
4–7.

Lawrence AM, Lewis L, Hofmeyr GJ, Dowsweel T, Styles C. Maternal Positions
and mobility During First Stage Labour Cochrane Data of Syst Rev 2009, 2. Art.
No CD003934. DOI:10.1002/14651858.CD003934.pub2.

Gottvall K, Allebeck P, Ekéus C. Risk factors for anal sphincter tears: the
importance of maternal position at birth. BJOG 2007;114(10):1266-72.

Dahlen, H. (2009). The relationship between maternal birth positions and
perineal outcomes in women giving birth in a birth centre over 12 years.Peri
Soc A & NZ 82.

Dahlen, H., Homer, C., Cooke, M., Upton, A., Nunn, R., & Brodrick, B.
'Soothing the ring of fire': Australian women's and midwives' experiences of
using perineal warm packs in the second stage of labour. Midwifery, 2009;
25(2), 39-48.

Caldeyro-Barcia R. The influence of maternal bearing down efforts during second stage on foetal well being. Birth Family Journal 1979a; 6:17-21.

Hofmeyr GJ, Hannah M. Planned Caesarean section for term breech delivery. Cochrane Database Systematic Review. 2003;(3):CD000166.

MacLennan A. Caesarean section does not reduce risk of pelvic floor dysfunction. British J of Obstet & Gynae.2000;107:1460–1470.

Roberts C, Tracey S, Peat B. Rates For Obstetric Intervention Among Private and Public Patients in Australia. BMJ 2000.15; 321(7254): 137–141.

Bamigboye AA, Hofmeyr GJ. Closure versus non-closure of the peritoneum at caesarean section. Cochrane Database of Systematic Rev. 2003, Issue 4. Art. No.: CD000163. DOI: 10.1002/14651858.CD000163.

Martensson L, Wallin G. Sterile water injections as treatment for low back pain during labour: a review. Aust NZ J Obstet Gynae, 2008; 48(4):369-374

Section 6: Early Post Partum

Thompson JF, Roberts CL, Currie M, Ellwood DA. Prevalence and persistence of health problems after childbirth: associations with parity and method of birth. Birth. 2002;29(2):83-94.

Spitznagel T, Leong F, Van Dillen L. Prevelance of diastasis recti Abdominis in a urogynaelogical population. Int Urogyn J. 2007;Vol 18(3):321-328.

Boissonnault J, Blaschak M. Incidence of diastasis recti abdominis during the childbearing year. Physical Therapy 1988;68:1082-1086.

Coldron Y, Stokes M J, Newham D J, Cook K 2007 Postpartum characteristics of rectus abdominis on ultrasound imaging. Manual Therapy. Epub.

Lee DG, Lee LJ, McLaughlin L. Stability, continence and breathing: the role of fascia following pregnancy and delivery. J Bodyw Mov Ther. 2008 Oct;12(4):333-48.

Viktrup L, Rortveit G, Lose G. Risk of stress urinary incontinence 12 years after the first pregnancy and delivery. O&G 2006;108(2):248-254.

Smith M, Coppieters M, Hodges P, 2007. Postural response of the pelvic floor and abdominal muscles in women with and without incontinence. Neuro Urodyn 26(3):377-385.

Wesnes SL, Hunskaar S, Bo K, and Rortveit G. Urinary Incontinence and Weight Change During Pregnancy and Postpartum: A Cohort Study. Am J Epidemiol. 2010 November 1; 172(9): 1034–1044.

Kearney R, Miller J, Ashton-Miller J, Delancey J. Obstetric factors associated with levator ani injury after vaginal birth. Obstet Gynecol 2006; 107:144-149

Haylen B. The retroverted prolapse: ignored to date but core to prolapse. Inter Urogyn J. 2006; 17(6):555-558

Bernardo M, Shek K, Dietz HP. Doesn partial avulsion of the levator ani matter for symptoms and signs of pelvic floor dysfunction? ICS-IUGA 2010 Toronto.

Slieker-ten Hove M, Pool-Goudzwaard AL, Eijkemans MJC, et al. Symptomatic pelvic organ prolapse and possible risk factors in a general population. Am J Obstet Gynecol 2009;200:184.e1-184.e7

Shetle M, Jones P. 2006. Effect of vaginal pessaries on symptoms associated with pelvic organ prolapse. 31stst Int Urogyn Assoc meeting. Athens, Greece 2006.

Whitcomb E, Rortveit G, Brown J, Creasman J, Thom D, Van Den Eeden S, Subak L. Racial Differences in Pelvic Organ Prolapse. O & G. 2009; 114(6):1271–1277

Wu W, Meijer O, Uegaki K, et al. Pregnancy related pelvic girdle pain (PGP), I: terminology, clinical presentation, and prevalence. Eur Spine J. 2004;13:575–589.

Albert H, Godskesen M, Westergaard J. Prognosis in four syndromes of pregnancy- related pelvic pain. Acta Obstet.Gynecol.Scand. 2001 Jun;80(6):505-510.

Thompson JF, Roberts CL, Currie M, Ellwood DA. Prevalence and persistence of health problems after childbirth: associations with parity and method of birth. Birth. 2002 Jun;29(2):83-94.

Norman E, Sherburn M, Osborne RH, Galea MP. An exercise and education program improves well-being of new mothers: a randomized controlled trial. Phys Ther. 2010 Mar;90(3):348-55. Epub 2010 Jan 7

Thompson J, O'Sullivan P 2003. Levator plate movement during voluntary pelvic floor muscle contraction in subjects with incontinence and prolapse-across sectional study and review. Int Urogyn J Vol 14(2):84-88.

Goodman J. Postpartum depression beyond the postpartum years. JOG&NN.2004.Vol 33;4:410-420.

Section 7: Recovery After Vaginal Birth

Dudding TC, Vaizey CJ, Kamm MA. Obstetric anal sphincter injury: incidence, risk factors, and management. Ann Surg. 2008 Feb;247(2):224-37.

Guise JM, Morris C, Osterweil P, Li H, Rosenberg D, Greenlick M. Incidence of fecal incontinence after childbirth. Obstet Gynecol. Feb 2007;109(2 Pt 1):281.

Matzel K, Manuel Besendörfer M, Kuschel S. The Anal Sphincter. Pelvic floor education .2008, Part V, 289-292, DOI: 10.1007/978-1-84628-505-9_36

Altomare DF, Ratto C, Ganio E, Lolli P, Masin A, Villani RD. Long-term outcome of sacral nerve stimulation for fecal incontinence. Dis Colon Rectum. 2009;52(1):11-7.

Wray CC, Easom S, Hoskinson J. Coccydynia. Aetiology and treatment. J Bone Joint Surg Br. Mar 1991;73(2):335-8.

Foye PM. Ganglion impar injection techniques for coccydynia (coccyx pain) and pelvic pain. Anesthesiology. May 2007;106(5):1062-3.

Section 8: Recovery After Caesarean Birth

Moore ML. Reducing the Rate of Cesarean Birth. J Perinat Educ. 2002 Spring; 11(2): 41–43.

What Every Pregnant Woman Needs to Know About Caesarean Section (Revised). childbirthconnection.org.

Dodd JM, Crowther CA, Huertas E, Guise J-M, Horey D. Planned elective repeat caesarean section versus planned vaginal birth for women with a previous caesarean birth. Cochrane Database of Systematic Reviews 2004,Issue 4.Art.No.:CD004224. DOI:10.1002/14651858.CD004224.pub2

Appleton B, Targett C, Rasmussen M, Readman E, Sale F, Permezel M, Vaginal birth after Caesarean section:an Australian multicentre study Australian and New Zealand Journal of Obstetrics and Gynaecology 2000. Vol 40(1):87–91.

Gregory KD, Korst LM, Fridman M, Shihady I, Broussard P, Fink A, Burnes Bolton L. Vaginal birth after cesarean: clinical risk factors associated with adverse outcome. Am J Obstet Gynecol. 2008 Apr;198(4):452.e1-10; discussion 452.e10-2.

Caughey A. Vaginal birth after cesarean 2008. Medscape emedicine.medscape.com/article/272187-overview

Section 9: Pelvic Floor Self Asssessment

Haylen BT, de Ridder D, Freeman RM, Swift SE, Berghmans B, Lee J, Monga A, Petri E, Rizk DE, Sand PK, Schaer GN; IUGA/ICS joint report on the terminology for female pelvic floor dysfunction. Neurourol Urodyn. 2010;29(1):4-20.

Fernandi M, Shek K, Dietz HP. Diagnosis of levator avulsion injury: a comparison of three methods. ICS-IUGA 2010 Toronto.

Orejuela F, Shek K, Dietz HP. The time factor in the assessment of prolapse and levator ballooning. ICS-IUGA 2010 Toronto.

Kruger J, Dietz HP, Botelho C, Dumoulin C. Can we feel with our fingers as well as we see with ultrasound? ICS-IUGA 2010 Toronto.

Burrows L, Meyn L, Walters M, Weber A. Pelvic Symptoms in Women With Pelvic Organ Prolapse. O&G: November 2004 Volume 104;Issue 5:(1)982-988 doi: 10.1097/01.AOG.0000142708.61298.be

Section 10: Caesarean Scars, Episiotomies and Perineal Tears

Liakakos T, Thomakos N, Fine PM, Dervenis C, Young RL. Peritoneal Adhesions: Etiology, Pathophysiology, and Clinical Significance.*Dig Surg.* 2001; 18: 260.

Lyell DJ, Caughey AB, Hu E, Daniels K. Peritoneal closure at primary cesarean delivery&adhesions.Obstet Gynecol.2005Aug;106(2):275-80.

Berman B, Valins W, Amini S, Viera M. Keloid and Hypertrophic Scar: Treatment & Medication. emedicine.medscape.com/article/1057599-treatment.

Baggish M, Karram, M, Anatomy of the vagina
http://www.urmc.rochester.edu/smd/gme/prospective/obgyn/documents/wk11d-AnatomyoftheVagina.pdf

MacLennan A, Taylor AW, Wilson DH, Wilson D (2000) The prevalence of pelvic floor disorders and their relationship to gender, age, parity and mode of delivery. British Journal of Obstetrics and Gynaecology 107: 1460-1470.

Section 11: Sex After Childbirth

Barrett G, Pendry E, Peacock J, Victor C, Thakar R, Manyonda I. "Women's sexual health after childbirth". BJOG 2000;107 (2): 186–95. doi:10.1111/j.1471-0528.2000.tb11689.x. PMID 10688502.

Brubaker L, Handa VL, Bradley CS, Connolly A, Moalli P, Brown MB, Weber A; Sexual function 6 months after first delivery. Obstet Gynecol. 2008 May;111(5):1040-4.

Rosenbaum T 2006. The role of physiotherapy in sexual health: Is it evidenced based? J Chartered Physio in Women's Health 99:1-5.

Barrett, G., Peacock, J., Victor, C. R., & Manyonda, I. (2005). Cesarean section and postnatal sexual health. Birth, 32(4), 306-311.

What are the risk factors for anal cancer? American Cancer Society. cancer.org/Cancer/AnalCancer/DetailedGuide/anal-cancer-risk-factors

Section 12: Return To Exercise

Smith MD, Russell A, Hodges PW Disorders of breathing and continence have a stronger association with back pain than obesity and physical activity. Australian Journal of Physiotherapy 2006; 52: 11–16.

Hodges PW, Sapsford RR, Pengel LHM (2007) Postural and respiratory functions of the pelvic floor muscles. Neurology and Urodynamics 26: 362.

Kramer M, McDonald SW. Aerobic Exercise for Women During Pregnancy. Cochrane Database Systematic Review. 2006;(3): CD000180. The Physical Activity Readiness Medical Examination for Pregnancy (PARmed-X for Pregnancy) csep.ca/forms.asp

Section 13: Birth and postpartum care in other cultures

The United Nations Population Fund http://67.205.103.77/about/index.htm

Elneil S. Vesico-vaginal & recto-vaginal fistula in the developing world. ICS News (5)2007. International Continence Society.

Sufang G, Padmadas S, Fenhmin Z, Brown J, Stones W. Delivery settings and caesarean section rates in China. WHO Programmes and projects, 2007;733-820. Bulletin of the World Health Organization. Volume 85:10

Hogan MC, Foreman KJ, Naghavi M, et al. Maternal Mortality for 181

Countries, 1980-2008: A Systematic Analysis of Progress Towards Millennium Development Goal 5. Lancet. 2010;375:1609-1623.

The Northern Manhattaan Study (NOMAS). Columbia University Division of stroke and critical care. columbianomas.org/study.html

Hold It Sister

the confident girl's guide to a leak-free life

Packed full of practical advice, case studies and recent research, Hold It Sister is a life guide for women to retain or reclaim their pelvic power.

'Every woman needs to know what's in your book – it is excellent and I highly recommend it.'
Dr. Christiane Northrup MD
Author 'Women's Bodies, Women's Wisdom' and 'The Wisdom of Menopause'

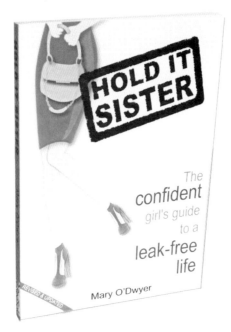

Available at book stores or www.holditsister.com
$24.95